Lynda AOUDIA

Chest X-ray

AF524564

Lynda AOUDIA

Chest X-ray

Techniques, indications, interpretations and semiological signs

ScienciaScripts

Imprint
Any brand names and product names mentioned in this book are subject to trademark, brand or patent protection and are trademarks or registered trademarks of their respective holders. The use of brand names, product names, common names, trade names, product descriptions etc. even without a particular marking in this work is in no way to be construed to mean that such names may be regarded as unrestricted in respect of trademark and brand protection legislation and could thus be used by anyone.

Cover image: www.ingimage.com

This book is a translation from the original published under ISBN 978-620-3-44614-2.

Publisher:
Sciencia Scripts
is a trademark of
Dodo Books Indian Ocean Ltd. and OmniScriptum S.R.L publishing group

120 High Road, East Finchley, London, N2 9ED, United Kingdom
Str. Armeneasca 28/1, office 1, Chisinau MD-2012, Republic of Moldova, Europe
Managing Directors: Ieva Konstantinova, Victoria Ursu
info@omniscriptum.com

Printed at: see last page
ISBN: 978-620-8-57039-2

Contents

Foreword

Thoracic radiography is an X-ray-based medical imaging technique. It is part of the daily activity of all practising physicians and is used in the routine assessment of all thoracic and/or extra-thoracic pathologies.

This book is not intended to be exhaustive, but our aim has been to put thoracic radiography at the forefront. This book deals with the physical basis of the formation of the radiological image, the different incidences of thoracic radiography and their indications, the different stages in the interpretation of a thoracic radiograph and the main radiological signs, all with the aid demonstrative diagrams.

This book is intended for medical students and practising doctors.

Professor Lynda AOUDIA

Chapter 1

Principle of X-ray image formation

1. Introduction

X-rays were discovered in 1895 by the German physicist Wilhelm Röntgen. He named the rays he discovered "X-rays" with "X" as the unknown in mathematics. The power of X-rays (Rx), which seemed marvellous, to penetrate opaque walls and reveal the inside of the human body.

In 1916 Wiliam COOLIDGE invented the X-ray tube known as the hot cathode tube.

2. X-ray tube

2.1. Definition

This is a hard glass bulb, unaffected by temperature variations, used to produce X-rays.

X-rays are electromagnetic waves (fig. 1). They are emitted when a beam fast electrons strikes a material obstacle.

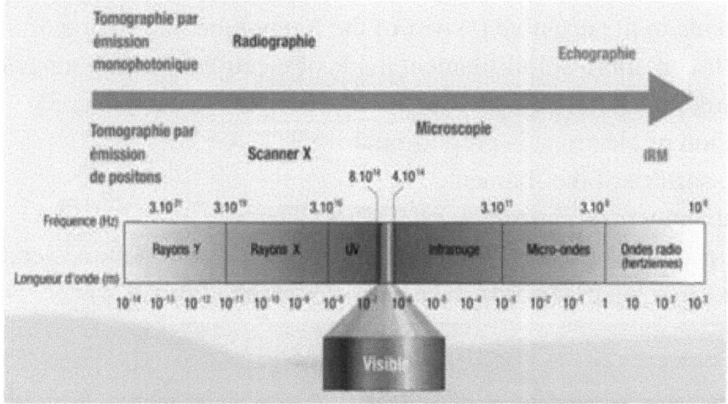

Fig. 1: Many of today's imaging methods use electromagnetic waves of different wavelengths and energies. X-rays are high-frequency electromagnetic waves that are invisible to the naked eye.

2.2. Description of the COOLIDGE tube

The X-ray tube or "Coolidge tube" is a glass enclosure with an absolute vacuum. It comprises (Fig. 2):

1- Two electrodes

- A cathode at negative potential (-).
- An anode with a positive (+) potential.

2- A cooling system (a lot of heat).

3- Two generators: essential for tube operation.

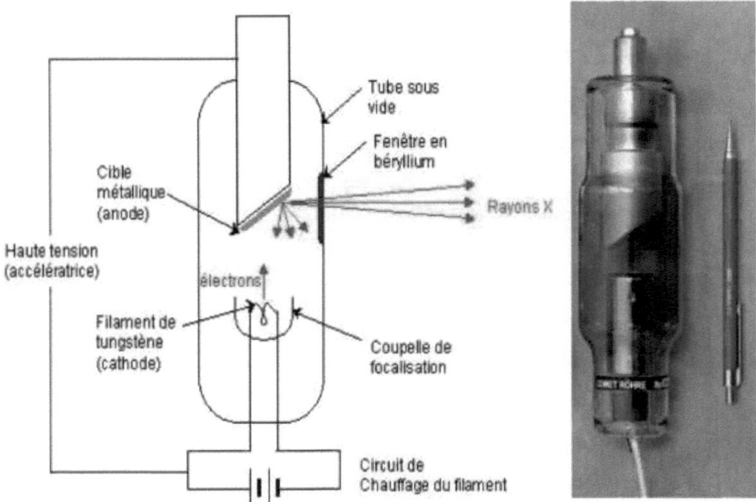

Fig. 2. x-ray tube

2.2.1. Cathode

It corresponds to the negative (-) part of the X-ray tube, the source of the electrons. It contains a spiral filament made of electron-emitting tungsten, heated to high temperature by a low-voltage current (10 KV) (fig. 3).

This emission of electrons is proportional :

- On the surface of the filament
- At filament temperature.

A high potential difference (PDD) between the two electrodes accelerates cathode electron beam towards the positive pole (anode) (fig. 4)

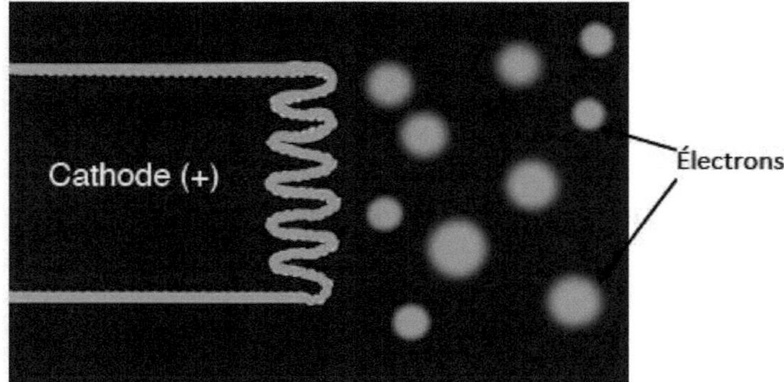

Fig. 3: The cathode

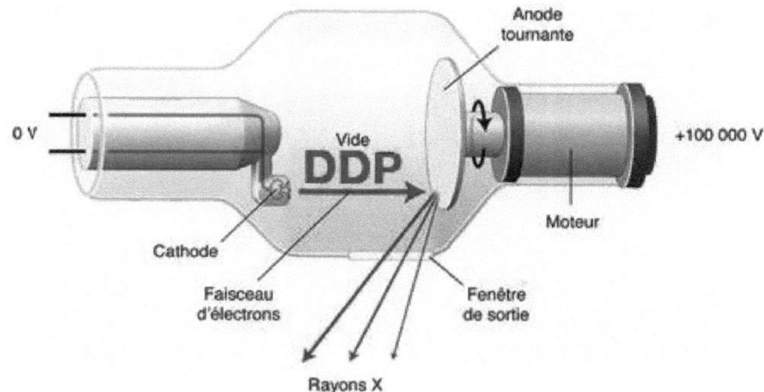

Fig. 4: Potential difference (PDD) established between the two electrodes.

2.2.2. Focusing electrode

Is at the same potential as the cathode whose role is :

- Repel electrons emitted by the cathode
- Avoid deformations of the filament caused by positive charges.

2.2.3. Electron beam (fig. 4)

- All electrons moving in a straight line.

2.2.4. The anode

The anode is the positive part of the X-ray tube and corresponds to the target. This is where the X-rays are produced, when the electrons, accelerated by the difference in potential between the two electrons, strike the anode. The anode is a disc-shaped pellet with a smooth surface, rotating at high speed from 3,000 rpm to 11,000 rpm (fig.5). The surface where the electrons are bombarded on the anode is called the focus and its size is a determining factor in the sharpness of the image (fig. 6). X-rays are emitted in all directions from the focus, but the X-rays are partially stopped by the anode itself. The greatest concentration of X-rays is therefore found in a direction perpendicular to the surface of the anode: this is known as a reflective anode (fig. 7).

The surface of the anode is at an angle to the direction of the electron beam to allow more X-rays to exit the tube.

The production of X-rays is very inefficient, since the yield in X-ray tubes around 1%. A large amount of heat is produced at the same time as the X-rays, which poses significant technological problems and limits, in any case, the quantity of rays produced. The anode is generally made of a tungsten-rhenium alloy because tungsten has a high atomic number (Z = 74), which favours efficiency, but also has a high melting point.

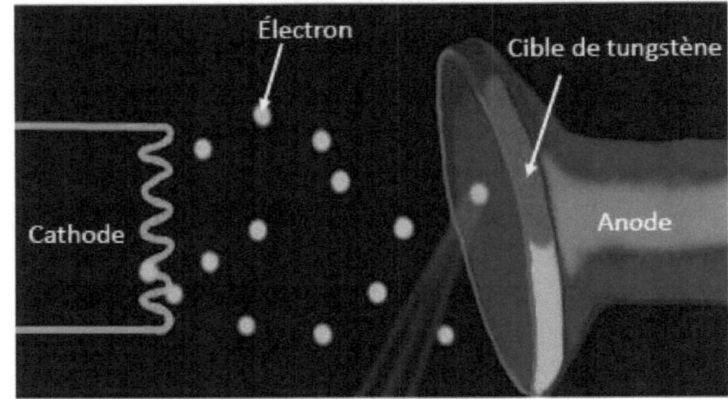

Fig. 5. anode.

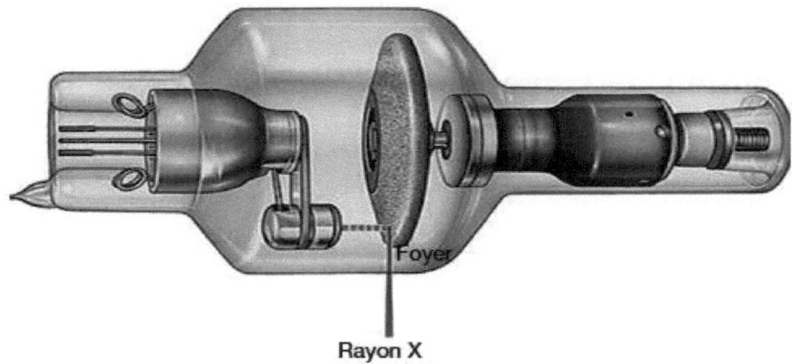

Fig. 6 Anode focus.

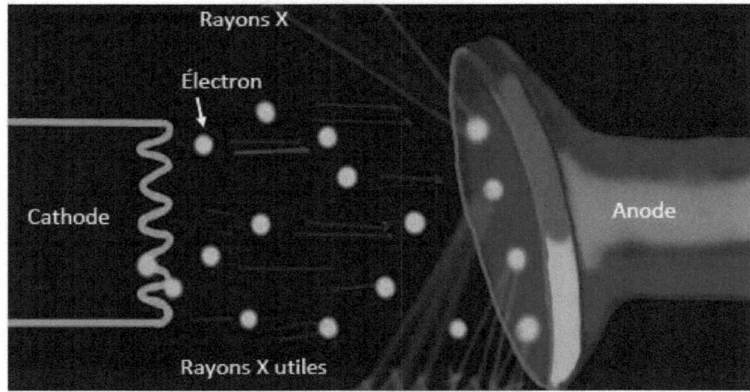

Fig. 7: Reflective anode.

2.2.5. Cooling system

Only 1% of the X-rays are emitted, most of which is heat (99%). A large amount of heat is produced at the same time as the X-rays and must be dissipated.

Overheating of the anode limits the electrical power (kW) that can be used to produce X-rays.

The advantages of the rotating anode :

- The home is constantly renewed.
- Spread the heat over a larger area.
- Increase the quantity of X-rays produced.
- Reduce the size of the firebox at low wattages.
- This improves the sharpness of the image.

2.2.6. Protective envelopes

The X-ray tube is surrounded by a number of protective envelopes to provide electrical, thermal and mechanical protection for the tube, as well as providing users with protection against leakage radiation.

2.2.6.1 Glass ampoule

Its function is provide electrical insulation, evacuate the heat produced and ensure as perfect a vacuum as possible. In the absence of a vacuum, unacceptable parasitic electrical phenomena occur (prevents interaction of the electron beam with the atoms making up ambient air). The bulb is generally made of glass (fig.8) :

- Good electrical insulation
- Allows heat radiation to pass through

Easy welding with metal electrodes

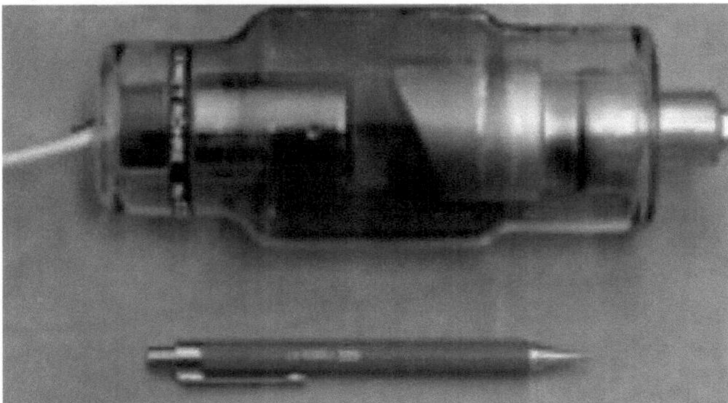

Fig. 8. glass ampoule

2.2.7. Lead sheath

The bulb is immersed in oil, which contributes to the cooling system. The whole unit is enclosed in a lead metal casing (fig. 9), ensuring :

1. Evacuation of the heat produced
2. Mechanical protection of the tube
3. Absorption of unwanted X-rays

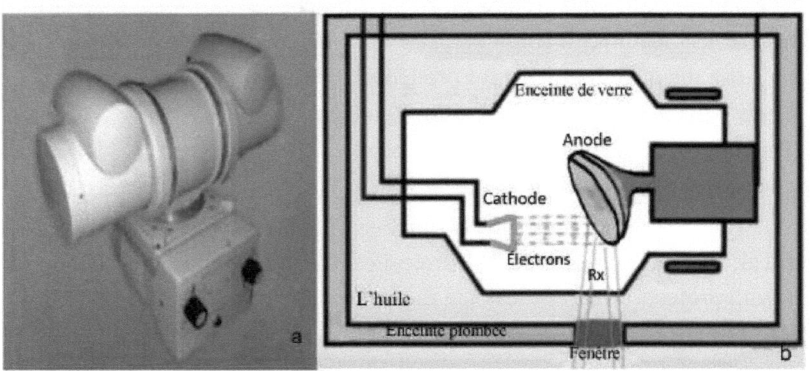

Fig. 9 Lead sheath (a) photo (b) diagram

2.2.8. Filter

Placed at the tube outlet, it eliminates soft rays and homogenises the beam.

2.2.8.1 Inherent filtration

The glass and oil in the tube stop low-energy photons that do not contribute to the formation of the image.

2.2.8.2 Additional filtration

The addition of a 2 mm plate of aluminium and/or copper also it possible to stop low-energy photons that are not involved in image formation (fig. 10).

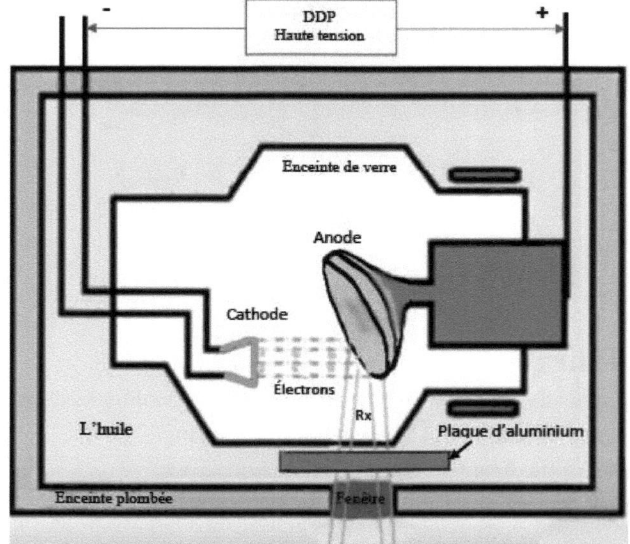

Fig. 10. Filter.

2.2.9. Diaphragms

Adjust the size of the radiographic field (fig. 11).

There are two types:

- Simple (square or rectangular field)
- Multiple: presence of superimposed diaphragms, the opening of which depends on the distance from the window.

Diaphragms to limit :

- The precision of the X-ray beam
- Scattered radiation

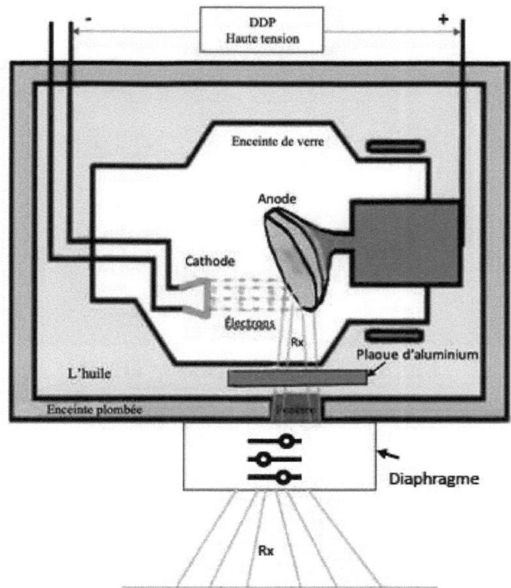

Fig. 11. diaphragm.

3. X-ray production

The X-ray tube or "Coolidge tube" is a glass enclosure with a high vacuum:

- A cathode at negative potential (-) and an anode at positive potential (+).
- The cathode contains a tungsten filament which emits electrons.

3.1. Mechanism

Electrons are produced from a tungsten filament contained in the cathode, which is heated to high temperature by a heating current (the thermoelectronic effect). These electrons, extracted from the metal, are then accelerated by an electrical voltage of several tens of kilovolts, which is maintained between the filament (cathode) and the metal target (anode or anticathode). These electrons collide with the metal target of the anode (braking effect) and their kinetic energies are transformed into X-rays and heat that must be dissipated.

3.2. Braking effect

The incident electron arrives at the target. It approaches the nucleus of an atom, which deflects it due to its positive charge, which attracts it. The electron is therefore slowed down. The braking energy is released in the form of an X photon or heat if the energy is low. The electron continues its journey along a different trajectory, having been deflected by the braking, until it reaches the next atom where it produces another X photon (fig. 12).

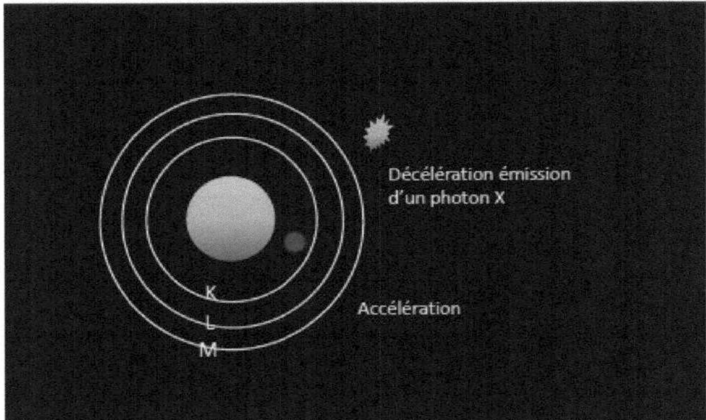

Fig. 12: Electron braking effect.

3.3. Properties of X-rays

X-rays are a form of electromagnetic radiation in the same way as visible light:

- Their wavelength is ($\lambda = 10$nm).
- They penetrate the body easily.
- They are easily absorbed by the air.
- They cause the elimination of certain mineral salts.
- They can have an analgesic or radiotherapeutic effect.

4. X-ray image formation

Three factors are essential for the formation of a radiological image (fig. 13)

- The X-ray source (F): source of the X-ray beam.
- The object to be radiographed (0): the object whose image is to be formed.
- The receiver (R): cassette containing the film.

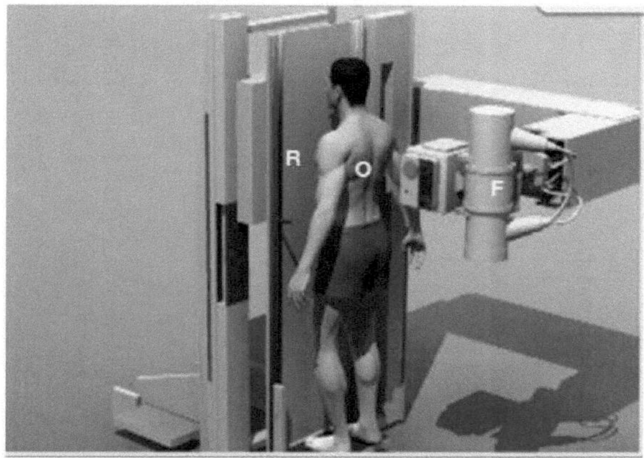

Fig. 13: Diagram of image formation. (F) X-ray focus (O) Object (R) Receiver.

When the X-ray tube emits its beam and it reaches the patient, three phenomena are observed:

- Some of it is absorbed by the organs in proportions that vary according to their density, resulting in the formation of the actual image on the film.
- Another part of the beam is scattered or deflected, causing blurring of the image. (This is increased in obese patients), hence the need for an anti-diffusing grid.
- A final fraction of the X-rays pass directly through the film, causing it to darken.

5. X-ray density

X-rays are absorbed to a greater or lesser extent depending on the substances they pass through. There are 4 radiological densities, from the most to the least absorbent (fig. 14):

- Calcic (very opaque): bone.
- Hydrous or liquid (opaque): blood, cream, etc.
- Greasy (not very opaque): fatty tissue.
- Aérique (clear): air.

Bone absorbs X-rays to a great extent, so it will appear white, which in radiological terms is called opaque. Air that absorbs few X-rays will appear black, which in radiological terms is called clear.

Any image that appears white on the plate is referred to as opaque and any image that appears black is referred to as clear.

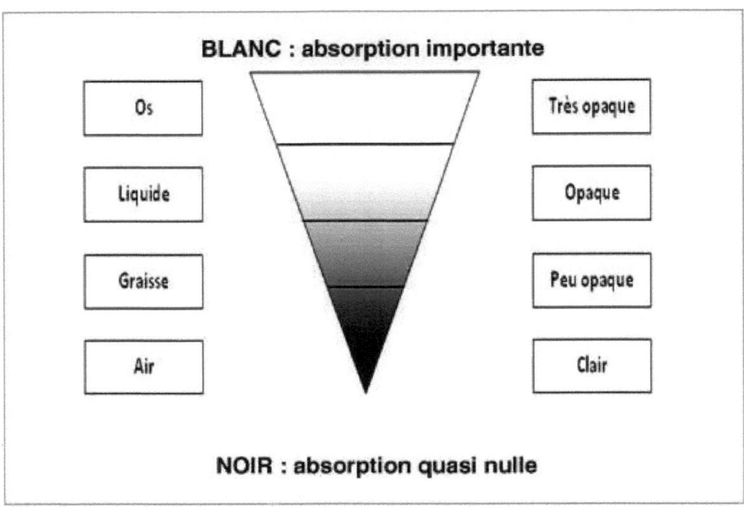

Fig. 14. Densités radiologiques.

6. Anti-diffusion grille

At the patient's exit, the scattered radiation can represent 5 times the direct radiation carrying the information. Scattered radiation alters the image. It is therefore essential to eliminate most of this scattered radiation; to do this we use the anti-scatter grid (fig. 15).

The anti-scattering grid is a large, thin plate made up of evenly-spaced lead strips. These blades allow most of the perpendicular rays to pass through but absorb most of the scattered rays. A small quantity of absorbed perpendicular rays is the cause of the grid effect. This effect can be avoided by mobilising the grid during exposure to radiation (the Potter system).

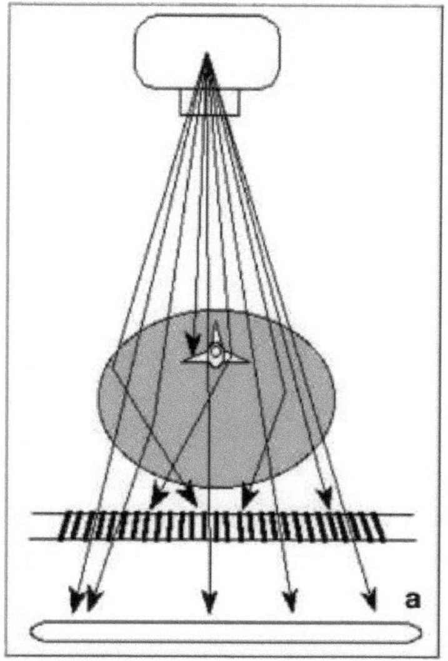

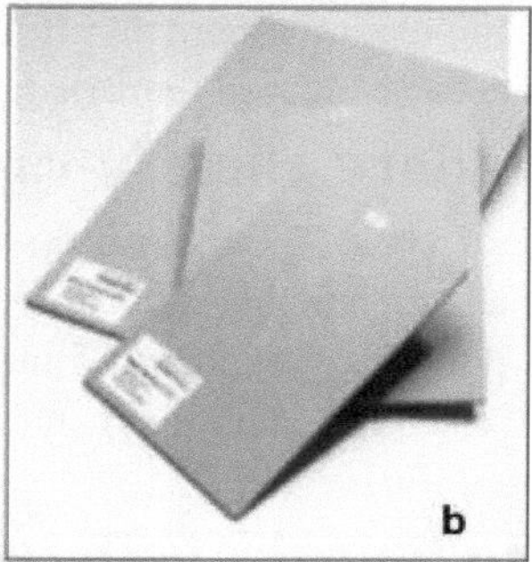

Fig. 15. anti-diffusing louvres. (a) Anti-diffusing grille operation. (b) Anti-diffusing louvres.

7. Applications in medical imaging

X-rays can be used in a number of areas:

- Standard radiography of the skeleton
- Chest X-ray
- Specialist examination
- Computed tomography

8. Contraindication

- Pregnancy

Chapter 2

Standard chest X-ray examination techniques

1. Introduction

At present, a chest film is still the essential first-line examination for any bronchopulmonary pathology.

Chest computed tomography (CT) and magnetic resonance imaging (MRI) should never be ordered immediately.

2. Standard chest X-ray

A standard chest X-ray is an essential part of any clinical assessment. It is a simple technique involving the use of X-rays.

Routine pulmonary exploration includes two views, one frontal and one lateral, as well as other additional views (oblique, lordosis, lateral decubitus or exhalation) if necessary.

2.1. Radiological effects

Routine pulmonary exploration includes two images, one from the front and one from the side.

2.1.1. Incidence from the front

- .1.1.1 Posterior-anterior incidence (fig. 16)

- Stand with chest against cassette.
- Deep breath.
- Freediving
- X-ray tube directed horizontally at a distance of 2 metres from the film, to reduce magnification and increase the sharpness of the image.
- High voltage (120-140 KV).
- Clear shoulders.

X-rays pass through the patient from back to front (Postero-Anterior)

- .1.1.2 Anteroposterior incidence (fig. 17)

- The patient lies supine or in a seated position, with their back against the plate (of interest in paediatrics or intensive care).
- Deep inspiration.
- The vertical x-ray tube, at a distance of 1 metre from the film (the image is enlarged and less sharp).
- Clear shoulders.
- The X-rays pass through the patient from front to back (antero-posterior).

- .1.1.3 Posteroanterior or anteroposterior incidence

Standing shots are preferable to lying shots:

- The lung range explored is larger (diaphragm lowered).
- The shot is taken more quickly.
- It's easier to achieve a distance of 2 metres horizontally than vertically, so the image is sharper and less magnified.

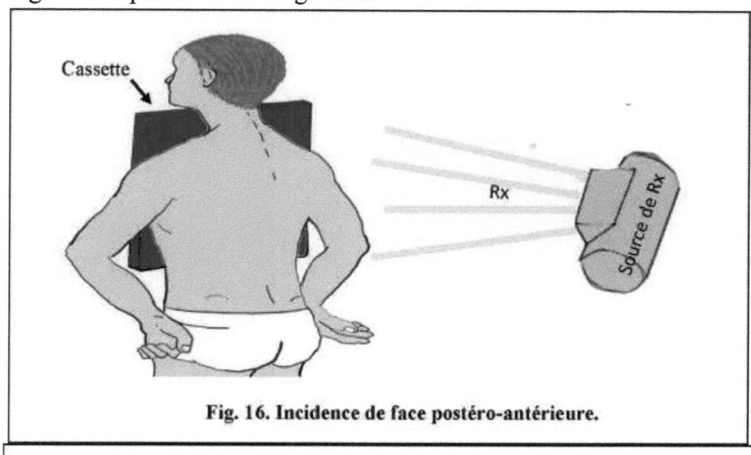

Fig. 16. Incidence de face postéro-antérieure.

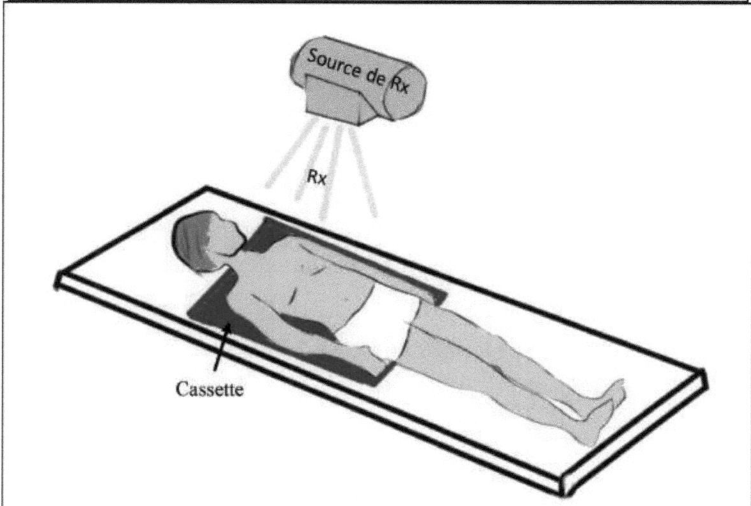

Fig. 17. anterior-posterior incision.

2.1.2. Incidence in profile (fig. 18)

- Standing position.
- Hemi thorax (right or left) against the cassette.
- Arms crossed above the head.

- In this case, the lesion to be studied should be as close as possible to the X-ray film.
- This allows the lesion to be located.

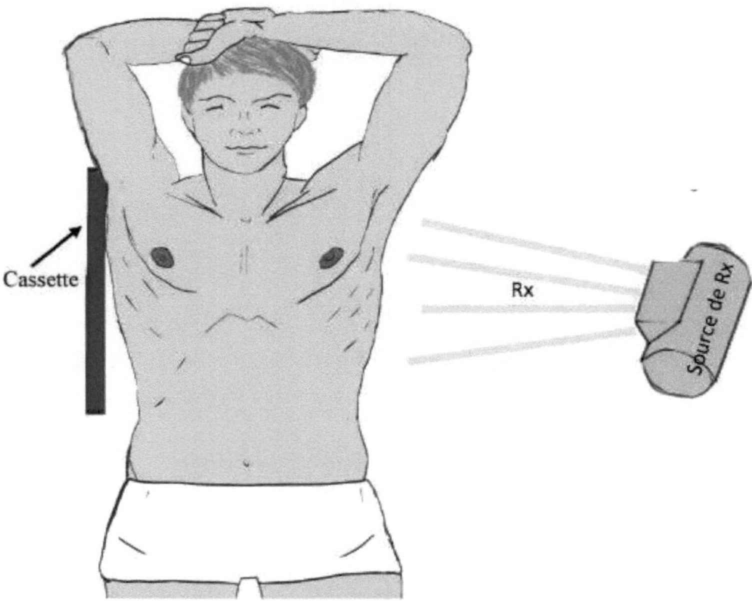

Fig. 18. Incidence in profile.

2.1.3. Other impacts

On request, depending on the questions raised by routine images. Less frequently used since the development of the scanner.

2.1.3.1 Incidence of expiry

Evidence of air trapping. Small pneumothoraxes and obstructive emphysema can be detected (fig.19).

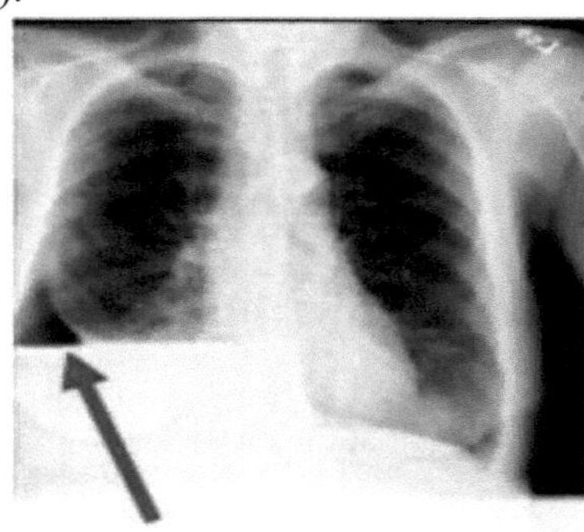

Fig. 19. Incidence of exhalation. Small pneumothorax (arrow).

2.1.3.2 Valsalva incidence

This is a frontal view, at the end of mid-breath, with the patient performing forced exhalation with the glottis closed. It can be used to determine whether a mediastinal opacity is vascular (its size decreases) or tissue-based (lymph node or tumour).

2.1.3.3 Oblique incidence

This allows lesions to be located and separated from superimpositions.

- To make a right anterior oblique incision, place the anterior part of the right hemi thorax against the plate (fig.20).
- To obtain a left anterior oblique view, place the anterior part of the left hemi thorax against the plate.

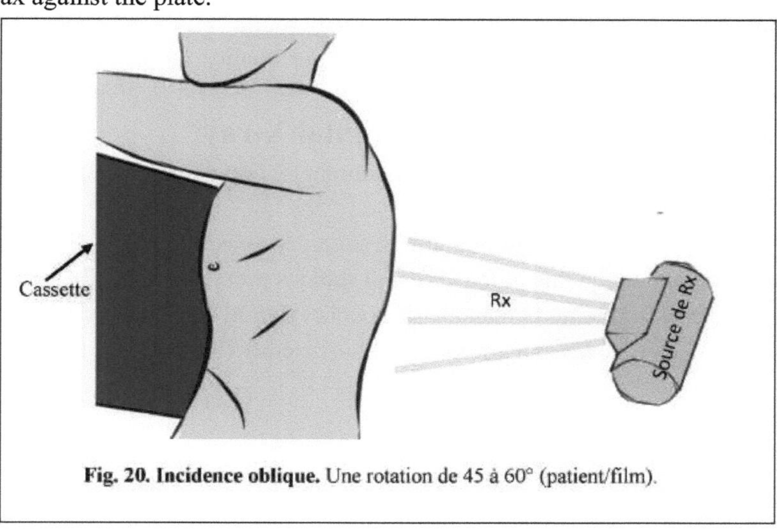

Fig. 20. Incidence oblique. Une rotation de 45 à 60° (patient/film).

2.1.3.4 Incidence in lordosis

The patient stands, with the radius passing from front to back (anteroposterior) and the tube elevated and tilted upwards at 45°. This angle of incidence not only reveals the lung apices and the foot of the lesser scissure, but also allows the middle lobe to be clearly seen.

2.1.3.5 Incidence in lateral decubitus position

Patient in lateral decubitus position, x-ray beam parallel to the floor. This approach reveals a small, free pleural effusion (fig. 21).

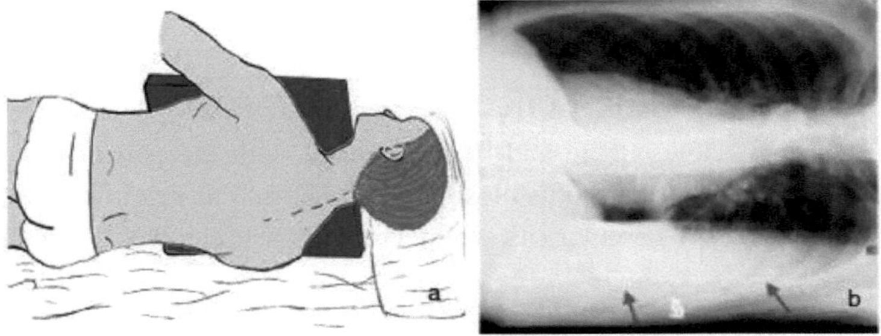

Fig. 21. Incidence in lateral decubitus position. (a) Patient in lateral decubitus position. (b) Liquid pleural effusion (arrow).

2.2. Quality criteria for a chest film

Only a rigorous technique produce satisfactory, easily reproducible images, ensuring effective follow-up over the medium to long term.

During any interpretation, a certain number of criteria, which vary according to the incidence, must be analysed to assess the quality of the image, before arriving at the actual analysis.

2.2.1. Criteria for a good frontal X-ray

- Identification must be clearly legible: surname, first name, sex, age, date and time the photograph was taken.
- The patient's face must be straight: in adults, the medial ends of the clavicles are symmetrical to the line of the vertebral spinous processes (fig. 22).
- The apexes and costodiaphragmatic pouches should be visualised (fig. 22).
- The shoulder blades and arms must be sufficiently free.

- The image should be taken with deep inspiration: at least six to seven anterior costal arches project above the right diaphragmatic dome.
- The photograph must be taken under apnea.
- In the upright image, the distance between the gastric air pouch and the top of the left cupola must be less than 1 cm.
- The image should be taken at high voltage, as a rule in adults, in order to obtain sufficient penetration of the mediastinum and moderate contrast. To judge that the image has sufficient penetration, vessels should be visible at the left base through the cardiac silhouette and the dorsal vertebrae at the top of the image.
- The plate must be correctly exposed, neither under- nor over-exposed. A print must be perfectly analysable on a light box without the aid a spotlight.

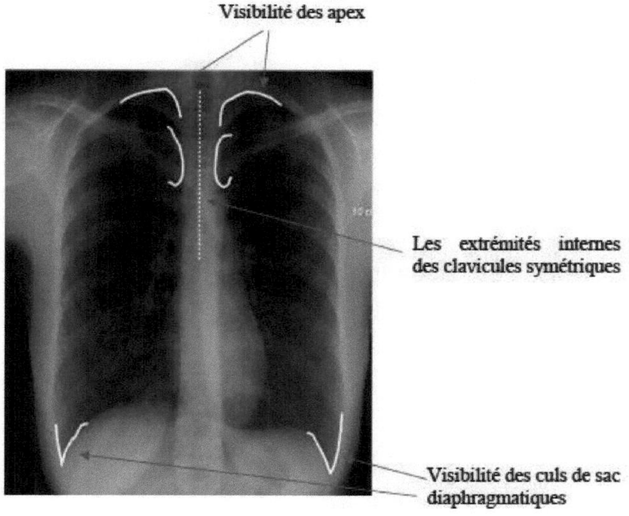

Visibility of apexes
Visibility of diaphragmatic cul-de-sacs
The inner ends of the clavicles are symmetrical

Fig. 22: Criteria for a good frontal radiograph.

2.2.2. Criteria for a good profile radiograph

- The identification must also be perfectly visible in all its elements: surname, first name, sex, age, date and time the photograph was taken.
- The patient's profile must be strict.

- The alignments of the posterior edges of the ribs are then approximately 1.5 cm apart, due to the difference in magnification of the two hemi thoraxes. If these alignments overlap, the patient is not in profile.

- Perfect profile of the sternum

- Grouped posterior projection of the scapular pillars.
- Good visualisation of tracheal clarity, the clear retro-sternal triangle and the clear retro-cardiac space (fig.23).

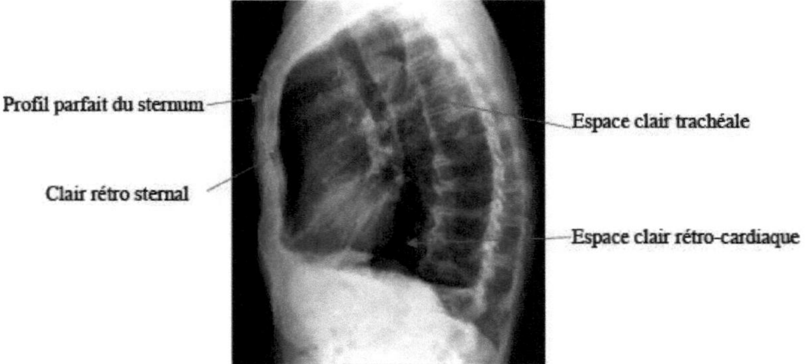

Perfect profile of the sternum
Retro sternal clear
Retro-cardiac clear space
Tracheal clear space

Fig. 23: Criteria for a good profile radiograph

Chapter 3

Lobar and segmental pulmonary anatomy

1. Introduction

Lobar and segmental anatomy is essential for interpreting a standard radiograph. The lungs are paired and asymmetrical, with the right lung being larger than the left. Lobar and segmental anatomy :

- Understanding pulmonary radiology.
- Locating a lesion.
- Prescribing drainage of a lung abscess.
- Identify bronchial orifices and extract foreign bodies by bronchoscopy.
- Segmental topography of certain diseases.
- Guiding bronchial fibroscopy, biopsy, surgery, etc.

2. Scissures

The lungs are covered by the visceral pleura. The pleura lining the surfaces of two lobes forms a septa and the space between two septa is a scissure (fig.24). The scissures separate the different lobes and are narrow spaces created by the folding of the visceral pleura.

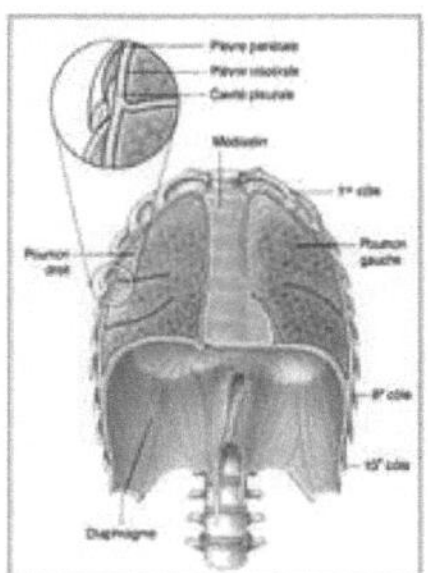

Fig. 24. Diagrams showing the septa and scissures.

2.1. Small fissure (horizontal fissure)

- Separates the middle lobe from the right upper lobe.
- Visible as a thin opaque line.
- Front and side views (fig. 25).
- Affects the lateral wall of the thorax, most often at the level of the 4th rib.
- Runs from the greater scissure to the anterior wall
- Absent in 25% of cases or incomplete.

2.2. Great fissure (oblique fissure)

- Separates the middle and upper lobes from the lower lobe on the right.
- Separates the upper lobe from the lower lobe on the left.
- Seen only in profile, from the front it is not parallel to the spokes (fig. 25).
- Oblique from top to bottom from the 5th dorsal vertebra to the anterior cul de sac.
- The fact that it is visible when viewed from the front indicates that one of its segments has rotated, which means that it is atelectatic.

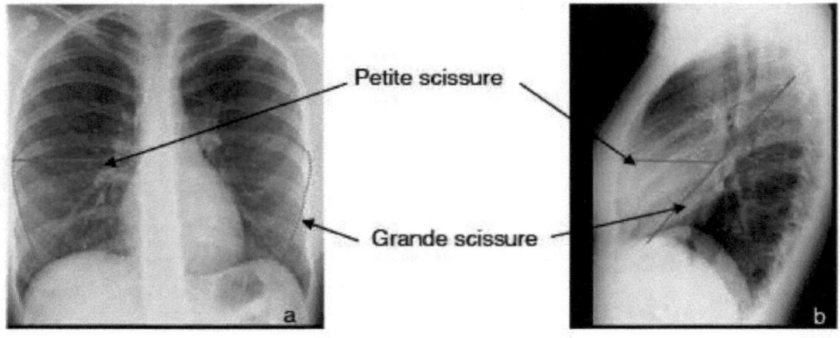

Small fissure
Large fissure

Fig. 25. Scissures. Standard radiograph: (a) Front (b) Profile.

2.3. Accessory fissures

2.3.1. Azygos scissure

- Formed by the joining of the visceral and parietal pleura by the azygos vein (fig. 26 a).
- Visible in 5/1000 cases.
- Located on the medial surface of the right upper lobe, it delimits the azygos lobe.
- Front view.

2.3.2. Paracardiac scissure (accessory inferior scissure)

- Separates a medial and basal portion from the rest of the lower lobe (fig. 26 b).
- Seen in 5% of cases.

2.3.3. Accessory fissure

- Separates the apical segment from the rest of the lower lobe.
- Sometimes confused with the lesser scissure, but in profile the lesser scissure is and the accessory scissure is posterior (fig. 26 c and d).

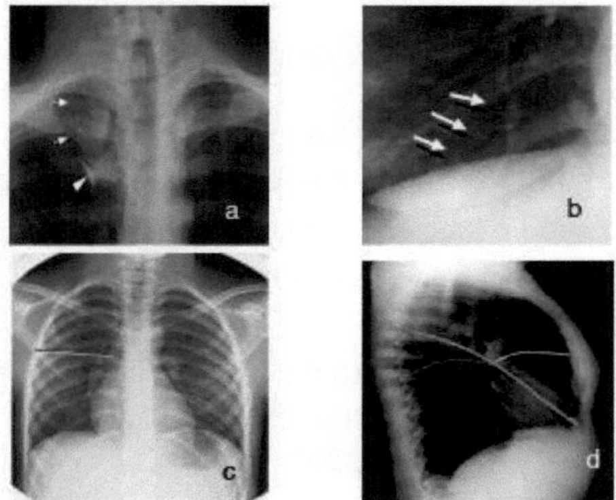

Fig. 26. standard radiograph: (a) azygos scissure. (b) paracardiac fissure, (c) accessory fissure in front (red). (d) accessory fissure in profile (red).

3. Lobar anatomy

3.1. Right lung

Consisting of three lobes (fig. 27):

- Upper lobe.
- Middle lobe .
- Lower lobe.

3.2. Left lung

Consisting of two lobes (fig. 27):

- Upper lobe.
- Lower lobe.

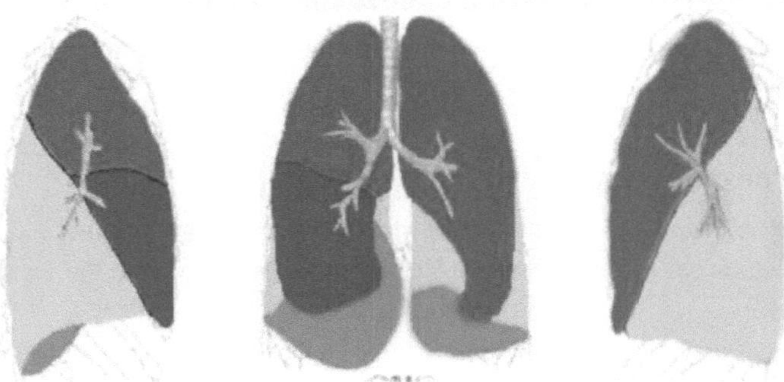

Fig. 27. Lung diagram: (a) Side view of the right lung, (b) Front view, (c) Side view of the left lung.
LS: upper lobe; LI: lower lobe; LM: middle lobe; GS: large scissure; PS: small scissure.

- Projection of the right upper lobe above the lesser scissure.
- Projection of the middle lobe below the lesser scissure.
- The right lower lobe projects completely into the lung field except for the apex (fig. 28).
- On the left, the 2 lobes project onto the lung field outside the apex, which corresponds solely to the upper lobe (fig. 28).

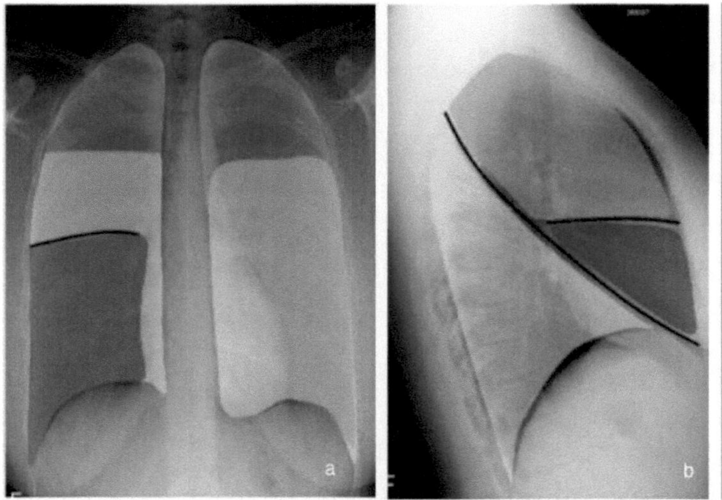

Fig. 28. Standard radiograph: (a) face, (b) profile. Upper lobe (blue), middle lobe (red), lower lobe (yellow).

4. Segmental anatomy

Each lobe is divided into segments by segmental bronchi (fig. 29).
The boundaries of the segments are more difficult to define because segmental

bronchi cannot be identified on a chest X-ray. We will simply describe the projection of the different segments on the front and side radiographs (fig. 30).

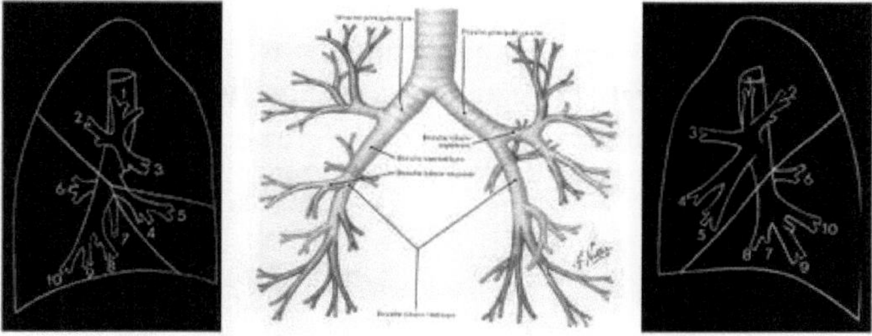

Fig. 29. Representative diagram of bronchial anatomy.

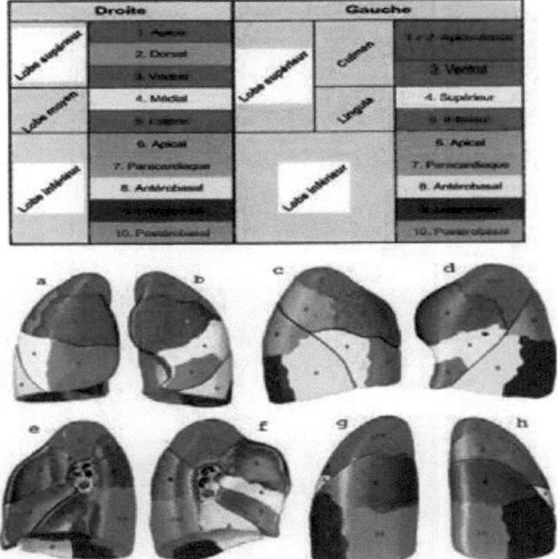

Fig. 30 (a + c + e + g): right lung, anterior aspect, external and internal profile, posterior aspect; **(b + d + f + h)**: left lung, anterior aspect, external and internal profile, posterior aspect.

4.1. Right lung

4.1.1. Upper right lobe

From the front, it occupies the upper part of the lung field. Its lower limit is represented by the lesser scissure.

In profile, this boundary is the upper part of the greater scissure behind and the lesser scissure in front.

Apical segment S1 (fig. 31). It lies flat against the mediastinum and is triangular with a hilar apex when viewed from the front and a median apex when viewed from the side.

Ventral (anterior) segment S2 (fig. 32). Triangular in shape with a hilar apex, it is bounded inferiorly by the lesser scissure and anteriorly and laterally by the wall.

Dorsal (posterior) segment S3 (fig. 33). From the front, its projection is similar to that of S2. In profile, its projection is triangular with a hilar apex, limited posteriorly by the wall and the upper part of the greater scissure.

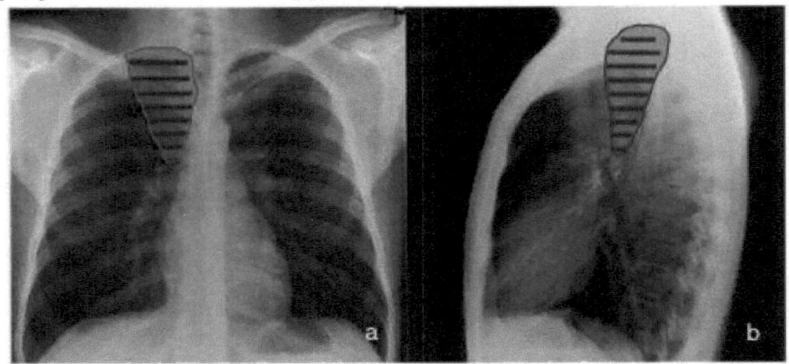

Fig. 31. Projection of the S1 apical segment. Standard radiograph: (a) face, (b) profile.

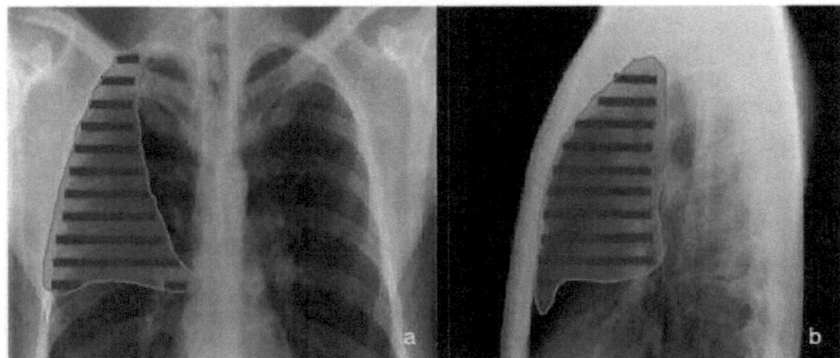

Fig. 32. Projection of the ventral segment S2. Standard radiograph: (a) face, (b) profile.

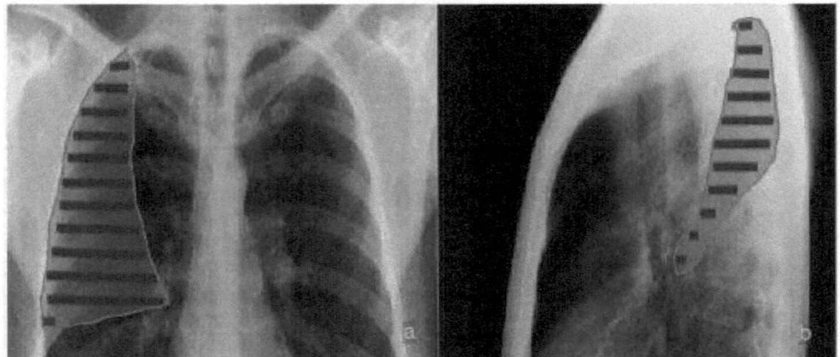

Fig. 33. Projection of the S3 dorsal segment. Standard radiograph: (a) face (b)

profile.

4.1.2. Middle lobe

From the front, its medial border is the mediastinum and its upper border the lesser scissure.

In profile, it is bounded by the lesser scissure above, the greater scissure behind, the diaphragm below and the chest wall in front.

Lateral segment S4 (fig. 34). Viewed from the front, it is limited at the top by the lesser scissure and has a triangular shape with the lesser scissure at its base. In profile, it is projected into the upper part of the angle formed by the greater and lesser scissures.

Medial segment S5 (fig. 35). From the front, it projects onto the right edge of the mediastinum, and from the side, it projects onto the lower part of the angle formed by the greater and lesser scissures.

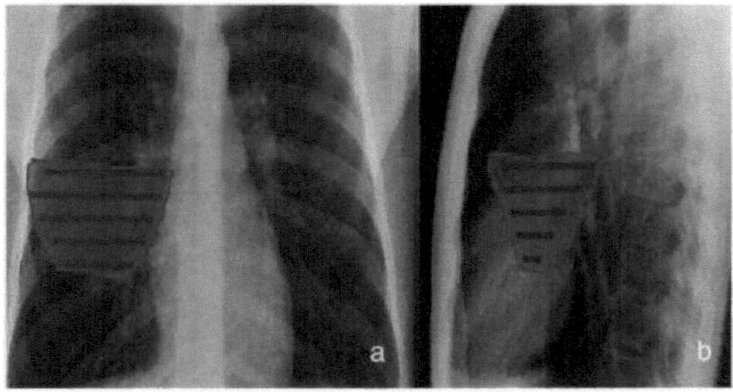

Fig. 34. Projection of the S4 lateral segment. Standard radiograph: (a) face, (b) profile.

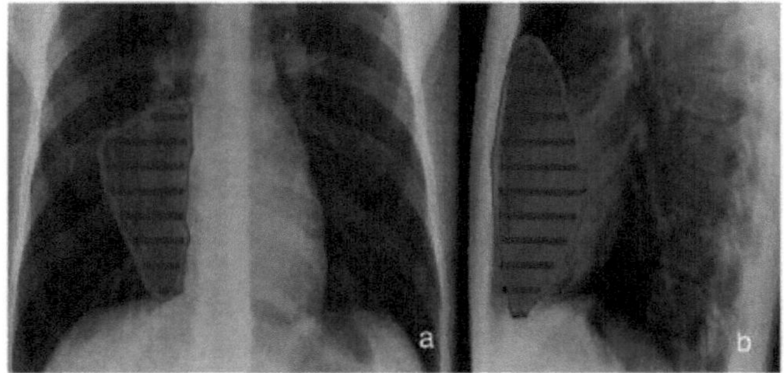

Fig. 35. Projection of medial segment S5. Standard radiograph: (a) face, (b) profile.

4.1.3. Lower right lobe

From the front, it projects over almost the lower two-thirds of the lung. In profile, its limits are represented by the greater scissure in front, the chest wall behind and the diaphragm below.

Upper segment S6 (fig. 36). It projects from the front above the lesser scissure, close to the mediastinum, but at a distance from the lateral thoracic wall. Its lower limit is close to the projection of the lesser scissure. In profile, it occupies the upper space of the angle formed by the greater scissure and the posterior wall.

The basal pyramid corresponds to the mediobasal or paracardiac S7, anterobasal S8, laterobasal S9 and posterobasal S10 segments.

From the front, S7 is juxtacardiac (Fig. 37a), S8 occupies the middle part of the lower third of the lung (Fig. 38a), S9 is lateral (Fig. 39a) and S10 is juxtacardiac posterior (Fig. 40a).

In profile, S8 is anterior (Fig. 38b), bounded by the greater scissure, S10 posterior (Fig. 40b) and S7 (Fig. 37b) and S9 (Fig. 39b) medial and superimposed between S8 and S10.

The anterobasal segment (S8) and posterobasal segment (S10) of the lower lobe are superimposed in front and in profile.

The paracardiac segment (S7) and the laterobasal segment (S9) of the lower lobe are superimposed in profile.

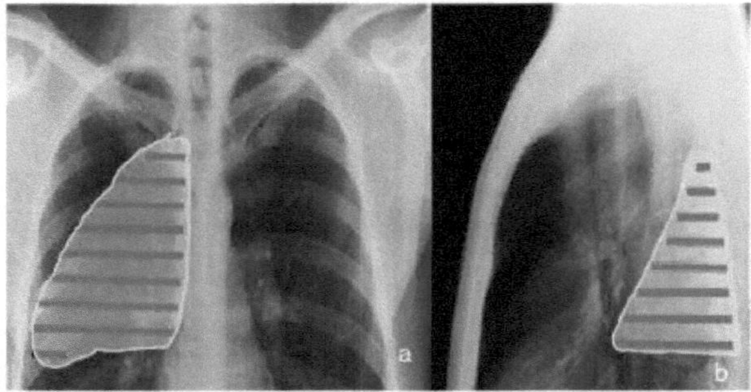

Fig. 36. Projection of the apical (superior) segment of S6. Standard radiograph: (a) face, (b) profile.

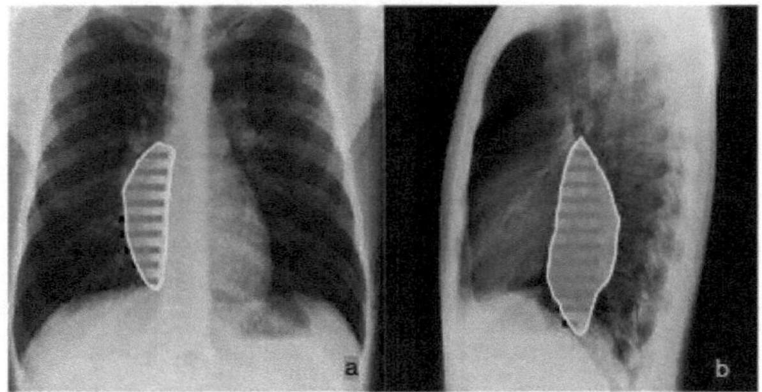

Fig. 37. Projection of the S7 paracardiac segment. Standard radiograph: (a) face, (b) profile.

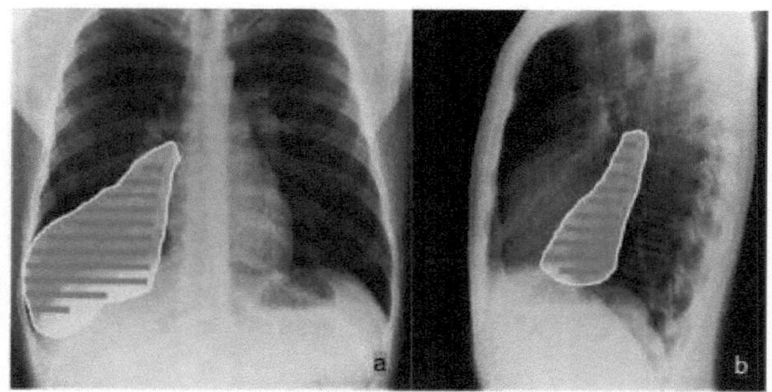

Fig. 38. Projection of the S8 anterobasal segment. Standard radiograph: (a) face, (b) profile.

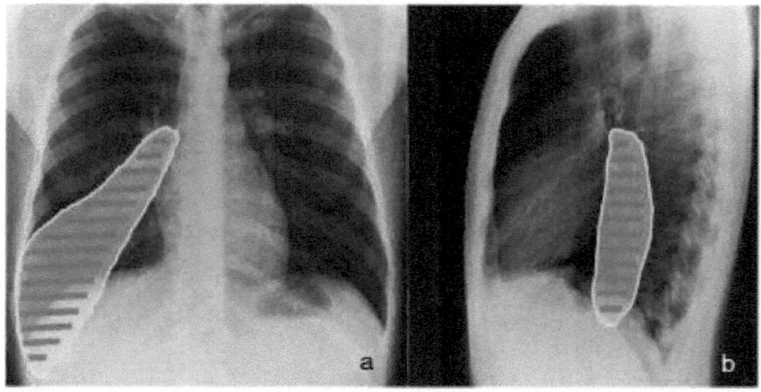

Fig. 39. Projection of the laterobasal segment S9. Standard radiograph: (a) face, (b) profile.

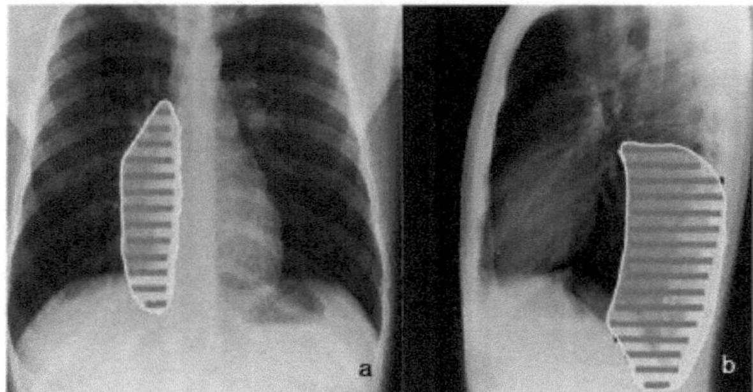

Fig. 40. Projection of the posterobasal segment S10. Standard radiograph: (a) face, (b) profile.

4.2. Left lung

We will not go into detail here as their projection is similar to that of the segments of the right lung.

Chapter 4

Interpretation of a frontal chest X-ray

- Always take the same approach to reading so as not to forget anything.
- The chest film is not limited to a study of the lung parenchyma.

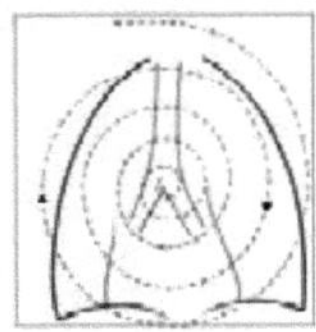

Spiral analysis :

- Patient's name, age and date

Quality criteria (fig. 41)

1. The dorsal vertebrae are clearly visible at the top of the image.
2. Symmetry of the medial edge of the clavicles in relation to the spinous processes.
3. The lateral position of the shoulder blades outside the lung fields.
4. Visibility of costo-diaphragmatic cul-de-sacs.
5. Diaphragmatic dome: below the posterior arch of the ninth rib.
6. Sufficient visibility of the vessels in the periphery of the lung(→).
7. The visibility of the vascular network behind the cardiac shadow .(→).

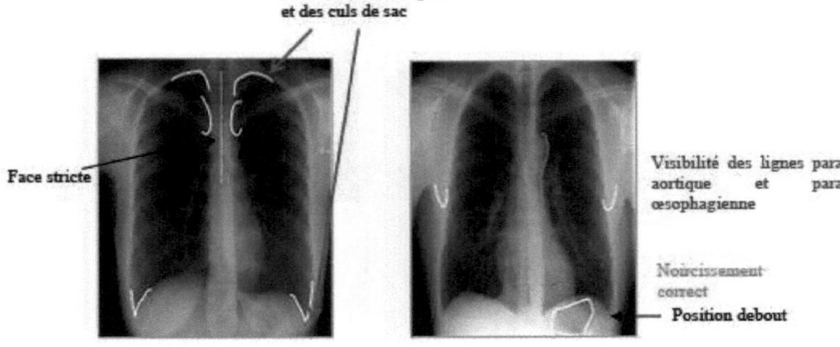

Visualisation of apexes and cul-de-sacs
Strict face
Standing position
Visibility of para-aortic and paraesophageal lines
Correct blackening

Fig. 41. Quality criteria. Standard frontal radiograph.

Analysis of the container

1. Soft tissue.

2. Skeleton (ribs - clavicles - spine - sternum).
3. Diaphragm and pleural reflection zones.

Content analysis

1. Lung fields and scissors.
2. Mediastinum: creur, bronchi and hilum.

1. Soft tissue

These are the least easily analysed elements, which can, in some cases, be confused with abnormal opacity.

Soft tissues from top to bottom: supra-clavicular hollows, axillary hollows, mammary glands (fig. 42).

The sternocleidomastoid muscles

Supra-clavicular hollows

Axillary lines

The mammary gland

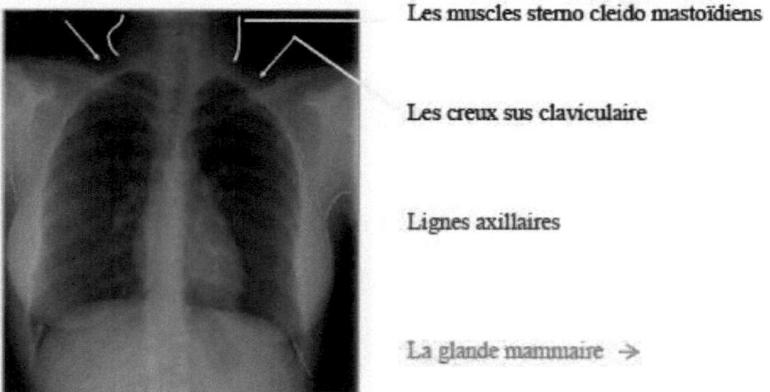

Fig. 42. Soft tissue. Standard frontal radiograph.

2. Bone structures

Los should not be overlooked, as bone masses or lesions can sometimes be found.

The bony structures from top to bottom: the clavicles, scapulae and humeral heads, the sternum, the ribs with a posterior, middle and anterior arch, and the vertebral bodies (fig.43).

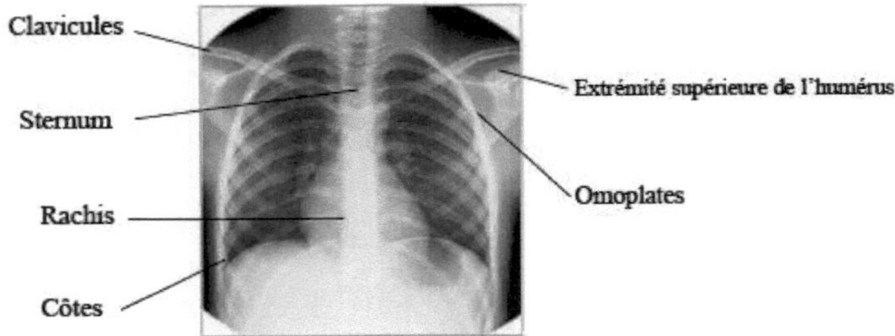

Clavicles Sternum Spine Ribs
Upper end of the humerus
Shoulder blades
Fig. 43. Seous structures. Standard frontal radiograph.

3. Diaphragm

1. The right diaphragmatic dome is 2 to 3 cm higher than the left (because of the liver) (fig. 44).

2. In young people, the dome is regularly rounded. In the elderly, it often has a fasciculated appearance.

3. The gastric air sac is visible 1 cm below the left cupola. Beyond this point, subpulmonary pleural effusion should be suspected.

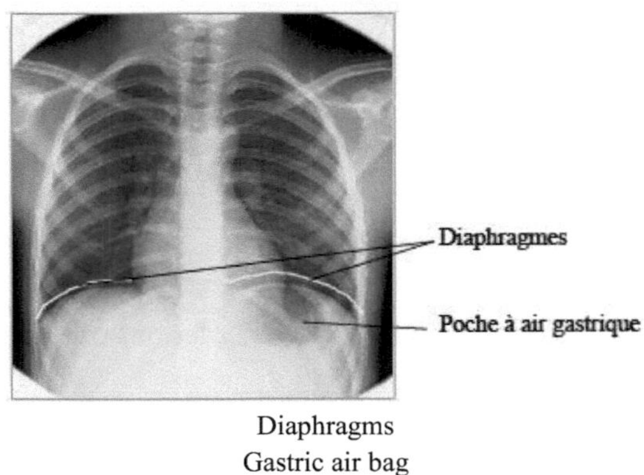

Diaphragms
Gastric air bag

Fig. 44. Diaphragms. Standard frontal radiograph.

4. Pleura

The parietal and mediastinal pleura, which is not normally seen except in pathological situations such as an effusion or pneumothorax.

5. Lung parenchyma

The lung parenchyma is made up of vessels known as "trabeculae", this trabeculae has a rather peculiar distribution, in fact the vessels will be wider at the base than at the apex, the apexes will therefore always look "blacker" than the base of the lungs, these vessels are visible up to 15 mm from the wall (information not used clinically). Nevertheless, these vessels are very important because it is thanks to them that we can detect a pneumothorax; under normal conditions they are visible, but if on an X-ray we do not see these vessels we must suspect a pneumothorax. We can also see bronchial tubes very proximally. It is very important to make a comparison between the two lungs, as this is how most abnormalities are identified (valid for all paired organs). Under normal conditions, there should be symmetry in the transparency and volume of the two hemithoraxes.

6. Mediastinum

The most important thing in lung imaging is to be able to identify the lines and edges of the mediastinum, which is what we systematically look for in order to identify any mediastinal mass.

6.1. The edges of the mediastinum

The border is formed by the junction of two structures of different density (fig.. The left side of the mediastinum is arterial and the right side of the mediastinum is venous.

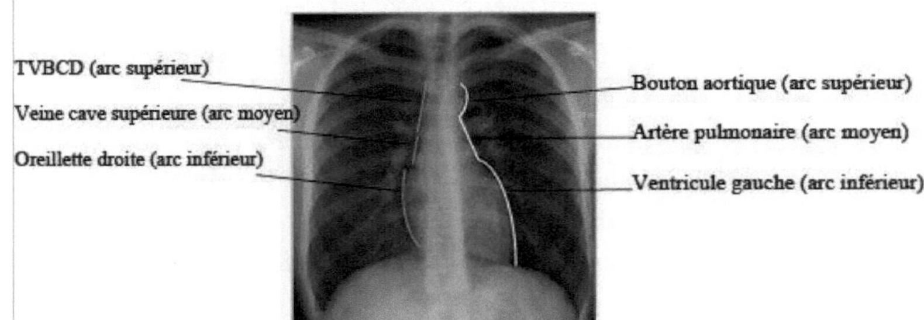

TVBCD (upper arch) Superior vena cava (middle arch) Right atrium (lower arch)
Aortic arch (upper arch) Pulmonary artery (middle arch) Left ventricle (lower arch)

Fig. 45. Mediastinal borders. Standard frontal radiograph.

Any deformation of these edges may be pathological. It is also important to take into account the patient's age: in a young patient, the aortic button is generally not very visible, whereas in an elderly patient it may be more prominent and calcified, known as an "unwound aorta".

6.2. Mediastinal lines

The line is formed by a fine structure of different density to the two neighbouring structures (fig. 46).

In practice: + lines form the mediastinal lines.

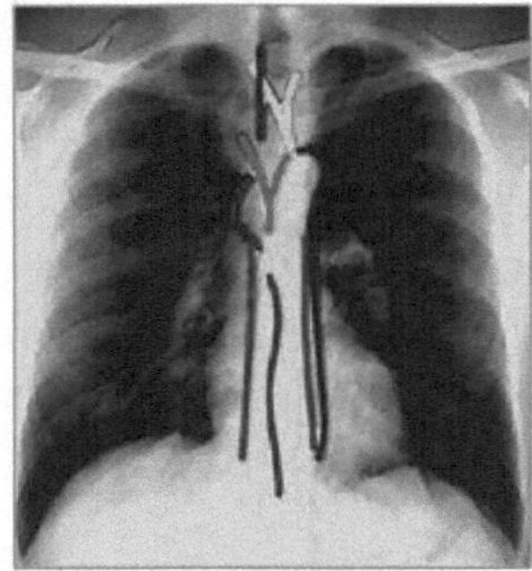

Anterior mediastinal junction line
Posterior mediastinal junction line
Paraazygoesophageal line
Para-aortic line
Left paravertebral line
Right paravertebral line
Right paratracheal band

Fig. 46. Mediastinal lines. Standard frontal radiograph.

6.3. Calculation of the cardiothoracic index (CTI)

It is also possible to detect cardiomegaly by measuring the cardiothoracic index. To do this, draw a horizontal line across the entire cardiac silhouette, divide it into two parts and divide the result by the thoracic diameter. If the result is greater than 0.5, there is cardiomegaly ($(a+b)/c > 0.5$) (fig. 47). Care should be taken not to diagnose false cardiomegaly in a bedridden patient who has had a recumbent X-ray, as the recumbent position virtually increases the size of the chest cavity and gives the illusion of cardiomegaly; the same applies to an X-ray taken with exhalation, which will give the impression of a large chest cavity.

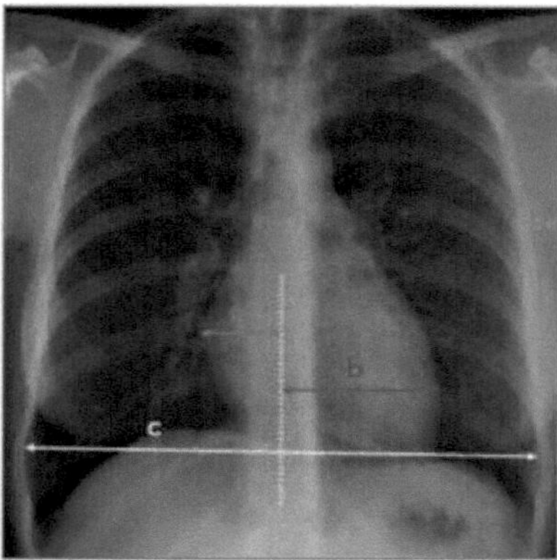

Fig. 47. Cardio-thoracic index Standard frontal X-ray. Measurement of the largest diameter of the right inferior arch (a). Measurement of the largest diameter of the left lower arch (b). Measurement of the largest thoracic diameter (c). ICT = (a+b)/c must be less than 0.50.

7. Lung hilar

The opacity of the hilum consists mainly of the pulmonary arteries and upper pulmonary veins; the lymphatics and nerves are not visible. The left hilum is higher than the right (Fig. 48).

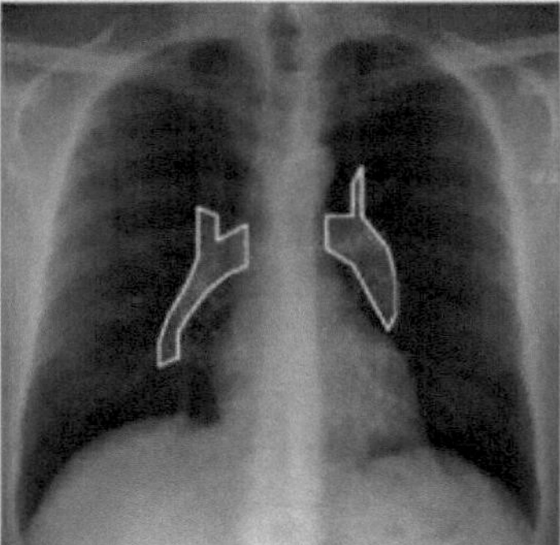

Fig. 48. Pulmonary hilus. Standard frontal radiograph.

Reading a chest X-ray: the steps involved

Administrative elements	Patient's identity, age and sex, date performed
Quality criteria for radiography	Symmetry, penetration, performed while standing and breathing in, full field of exploration
Image analysis	Step by step, systematic
1. Soft tissue	• Axillary hollows and neck: subcutaneous emphysema, cervical ribs • Breast shadows in women: asymmetry

2. Bone frame	• Fracture line • Lytic lesion • Surgical sequelae
3. Diaphragm and subdiaphragmatic organs	- Collapse or ascension of a dome, pneumoperitoneum
4. Pleura	• Fluid or gas effusion • Thickening and calcifications
5. Parenchyma	• Opacity: nodules, alveolar/bronchial/interstitial syndrome. • Hyperclartes: localised or diffuse
6. Mediastinum	• Mediastinal opacity or hyperclarity, aerated water level • Deformation of the mediastinal borders • Deformation of the mediastinal silhouette • Tracheal anomaly • Cardiomegaly
7. Hiles	• Hilar ascension: atelectasis • Hilar filling : Adenopathy

Chapter 5

Silhouette signs

1. Introduction

The silhouette sign is a fundamental sign in the interpretation of a thoracic radiology image. It is of great value in determining the topography of a lung parenchymal opacity, a mediastinal mass or an encysted pleural effusion.

2. Definition of silhouette sign

2.1. Definition (1)

If two opacities with a hydrous tone are located in contact with each other, and the ray is tangent to their interface, then their respective limits disappear at the level of the contact.

2.2. Definition (2) "Felson

A lesion opacity corresponds to that of water, in anatomical contact with the creur, aorta and/or diaphragm, will erase their contour along the contact zone.

2.3. Silhouette sign in practice

If two opacities, with a watery tone, merge together "a positive silhouette sign" (fig. 49).

If two water-toned opacities do not blend together, "a sign of the negative silhouette" (fig. 49).

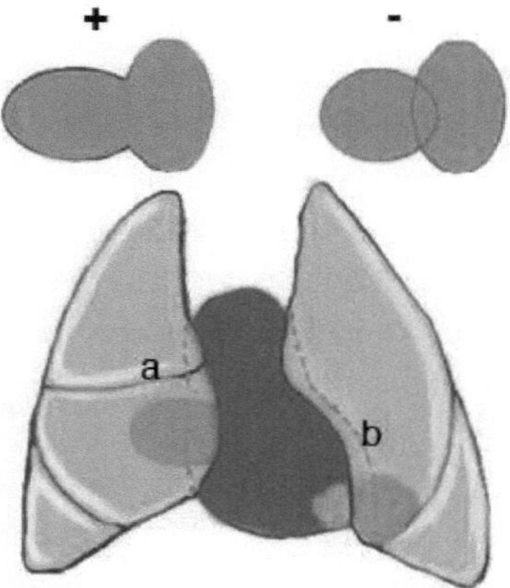

Fig. 49. Diagram illustrating the silhouette sign. (a) Silhouette sign (+). (b) Silhouette (-).

3. Interest in the silhouette sign

This sign is found at the cardiac and aortic interfaces.
It is of great value in determining the topography of an intrathoracic opacity, whether mediastinal, pulmonary or pleural.

4. Applications to lung opacities

- Intraparenchymal opacity, a watery opacity with an acute connection angle ($< 90^0$) (fig. 50).

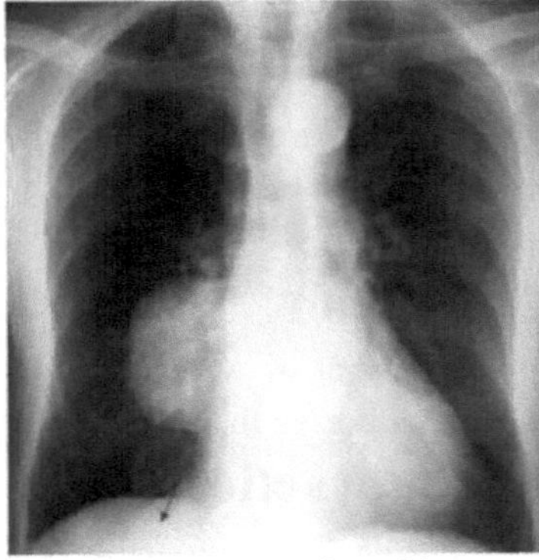

Fig. 50. Intraparenchymal opacity. Watery opacity, with an acute connection angle.

- A lung opacity that obliterates the right edge of the creur indicates that this lesion is located in the middle lobe (fig.51).
- A pulmonary opacity that does not erase the right edge of the creur indicates that this lesion is located in the right lower lobe (fig. 52).
- A pulmonary opacity that obliterates the left edge of the creur indicates that this lesion is located in the lingula (fig. 53).
- A pulmonary opacity that does not erase the left edge of the creur indicates that this lesion is located in the left lower lobe (fig. 54).
- A pulmonary opacity that obliterates the upper right edge of the creur and/or the ascending aorta indicates that the lesion is located in the anterior segment of the right upper lobe.
- A pulmonary opacity that obliterates the upper left edge of the creur indicates that the lesion is located in the anterior segment of the upper left lobe.
- A pulmonary opacity that obliterates the aortic button indicates that this lesion is located posterior to the apico-dorsal segment of the left upper lobe (fig. 55).
- A localised opacity at the LIG obliterates the descending aorta along the contact zone.

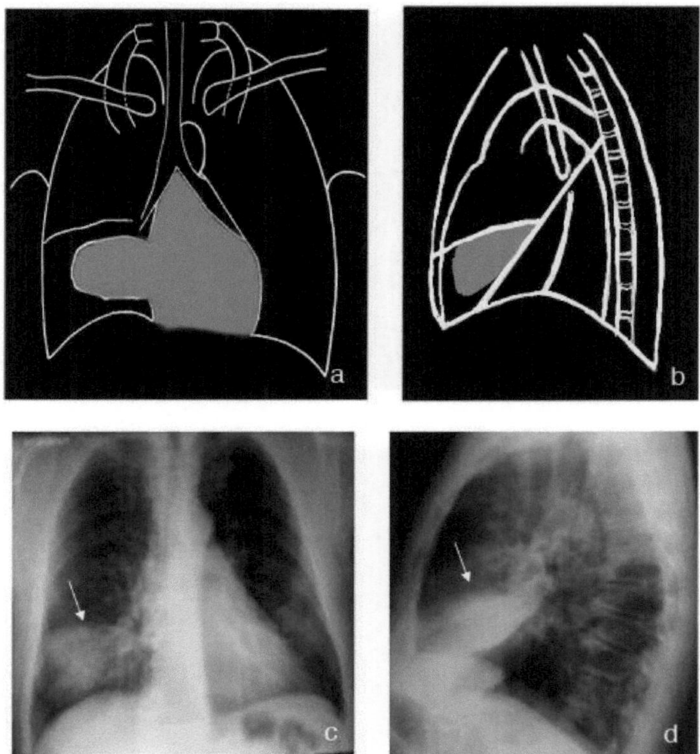

Fig. 51. Intraparenchymal opacity of the middle lobe obscuring the right border of the heart "positive silhouette sign" (arrows). Diagrams. (a) Front view. (b) Side view. Standard X-ray (c) front (d) profile.

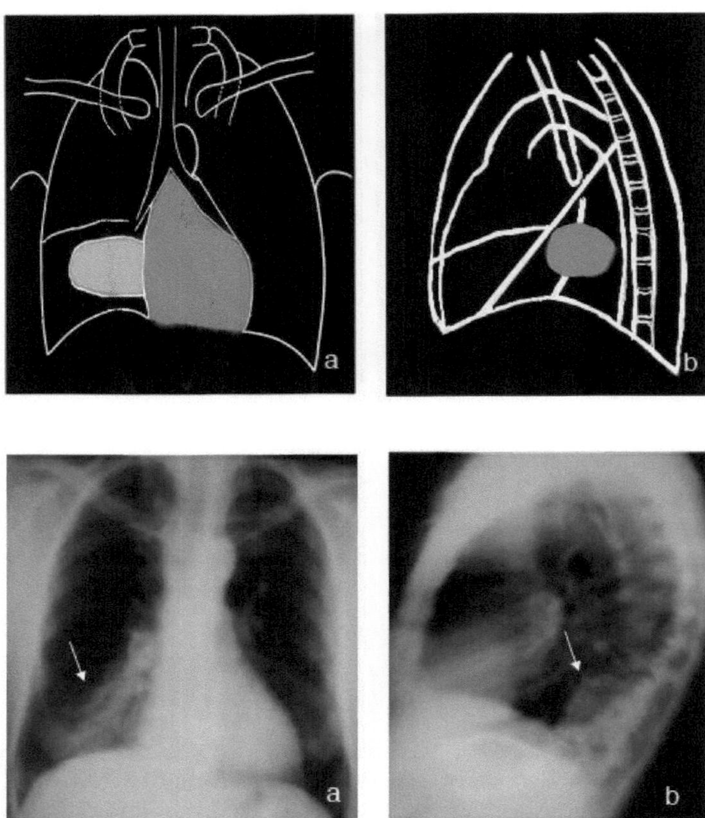

Fig. 52. Intraparenchymal opacity of the right lower lobe not obliterating the border right side of the heart "negative silhouette sign" (arrows). Diagrams. (a) Front view. (b) Side view. Standard X-ray (c) front (d) profile

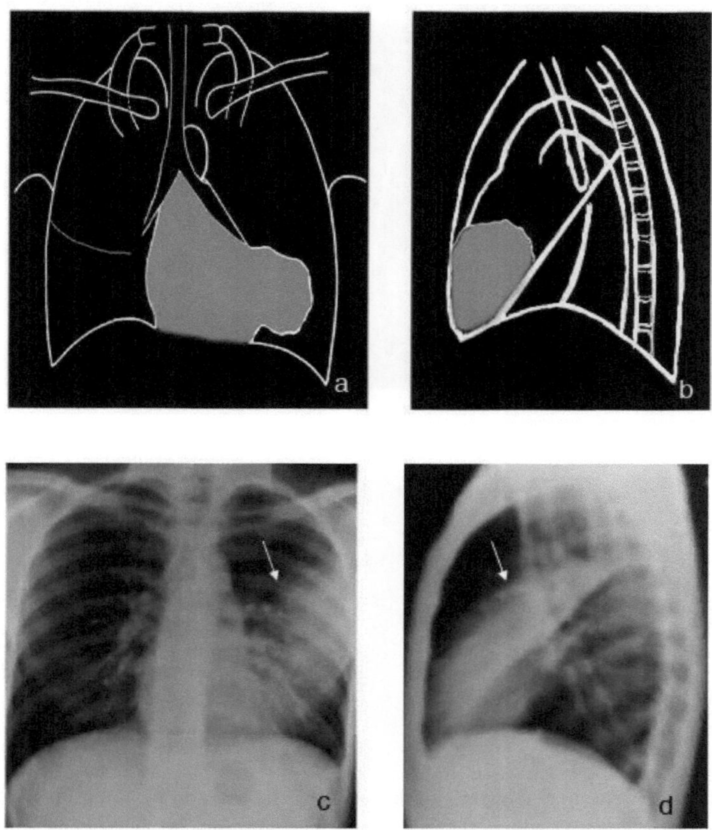

Fig. 53: Intra-parenchymal opacity of the lingula obliterating the left edge of the heart. "Positive silhouette sign (arrows). Diagrams. (a) Front view. (b) Side view. Standard X-ray (c) front (d) profile.

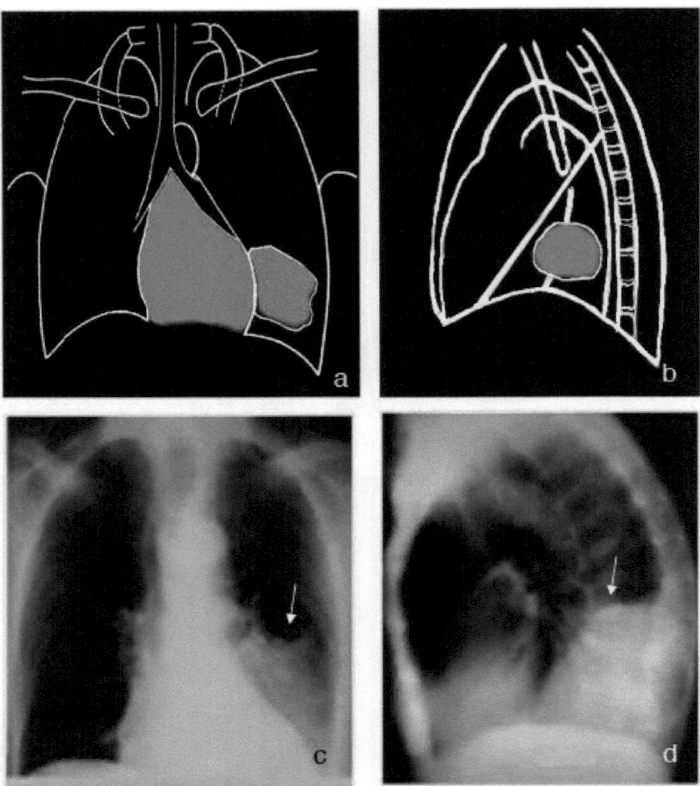

Fig. 54. Intraparenchymal opacity of the left lower lobe not obliterating the left border of the heart "negative silhouette sign" (arrows). Diagrams. (a) Front view. (b) Front view.
in profile. Standard radiograph (c) front (d) profile.

5. Applications to mediastinal masses

- Mediastinal opacity, an opacity of watery tone, with an obtuse connection angle with the edges of the mediastinum (> 90^0) (fig. 56).
- A mass in the anterior mediastinum obliterates the edge of the creur at its point of contact (fig. 57).
- A mass in the posterior mediastinum obliterates the aortic button at its point of contact (fig. 58).

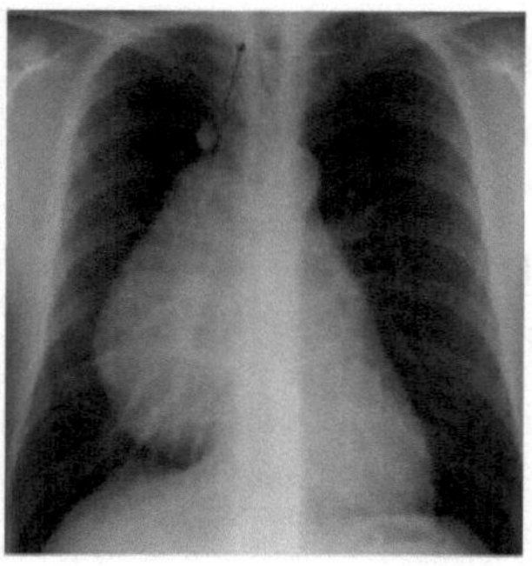

Fig. 56. Extraparenchymal opacity. Watery opacity, with an obtuse connection angle with the edges of the mediastinum.

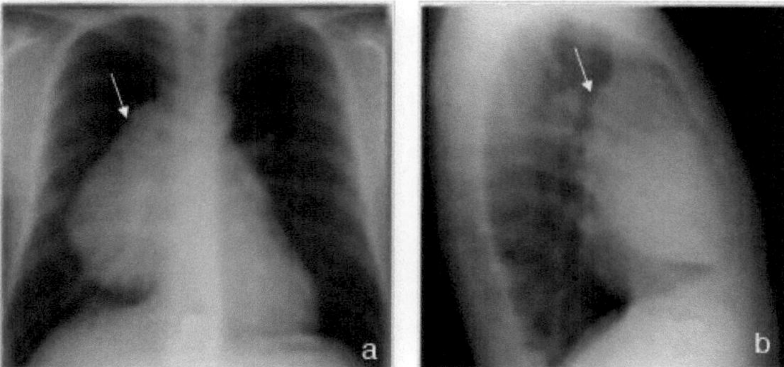

Fig. 57. Mediastinal opacity obliterating the right border of the heart "positive silhouette sign" (arrows). Standard radiograph: (a) face (b) profile.

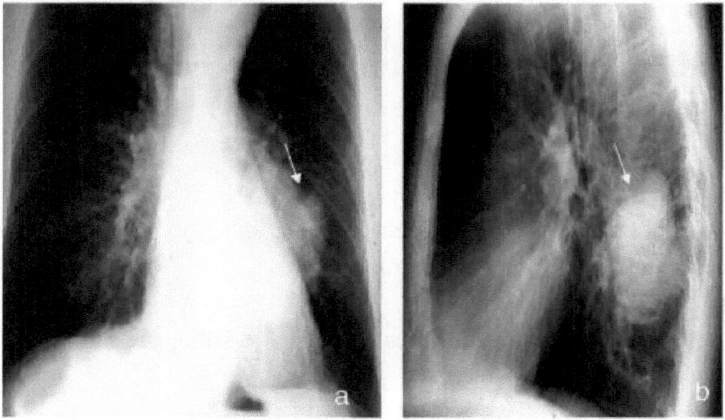

Fig. 58. Mediastinal opacity not obliterating the left edge of the heart "negative silhouette sign" (arrows). Standard radiograph: (a) face (b) profile.

6. Applications to pleural effusions

An encysted effusion from the anterior pleural cavity obliterates the edges of the creur or the ascending aorta along the contact zone.

7. Differential diagnosis

7.1. Physiological silhouette sign

The left diaphragmatic dome loses its silhouette in its anterior part, in contact with the creur (fig. 59).

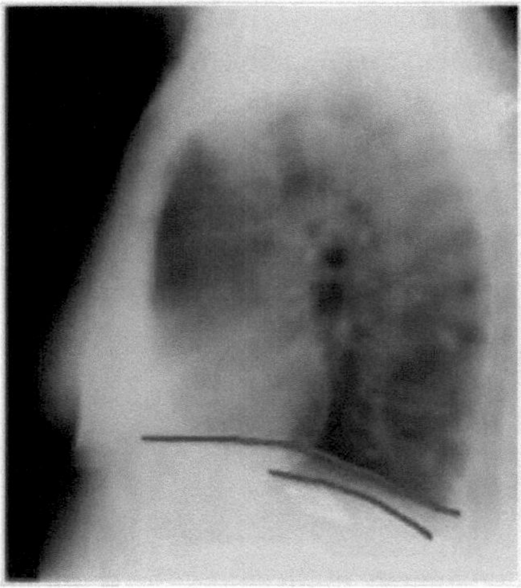

Fig. 59. The left diaphragm loses its silhouette in the anterior part, in contact with the creur. Standard profile X-ray.

7.2. Silhouette sign in a normal subject

The greasy fringe that erases the edge of the hollow.

8. Limits

The silhouette sign cannot be applied:

- If the right edge of the creur projects onto the spine.
- Patients with a funnel-shaped thorax.
- If the film is underexposed.
- Calcified lesions and areal cavities do not give a silhouette sign, as they have a different radiological tone in water.

Chapter 6

Aerated bronchogram

1. Introduction

In the chest X-ray, the intrapulmonary bronchi are not visible on a normal telethorax because they have very thin walls, contain air and are surrounded by air from the alveoli.

Only the pulmonary vessels are visible in the form branching arborisations extending from the pulmonary hilum.

2. Definition

The visibility of intra-bronchial air, underlined by the opacity of the alveolar filling in the distal air spaces surrounding the bronchi, defines the aeric bronchogram (fig. 60). This appears as a tubular clarity which bifurcates to form bronchi of normal calibre. When the bronchus is viewed from the front, the aerotic bronchogram appears as a rounded, well-limited clearness. Some segmental or sub-segmental bronchi with an anterior-posterior or posterior-anterior course can be recognised on a frontal view.

When present, the aerated bronchogram sign indicates lung involvement in the vast majority of cases.

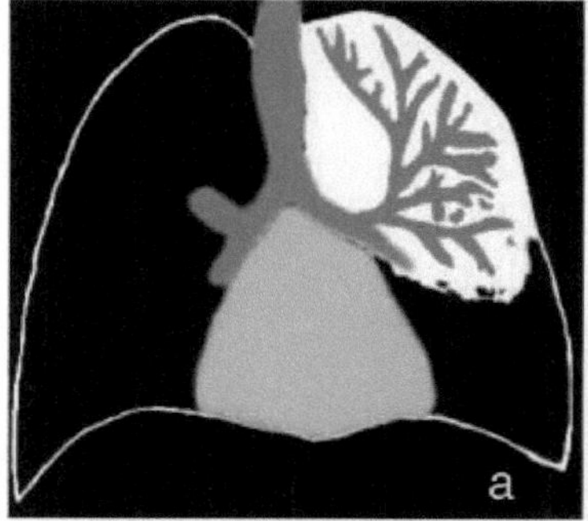

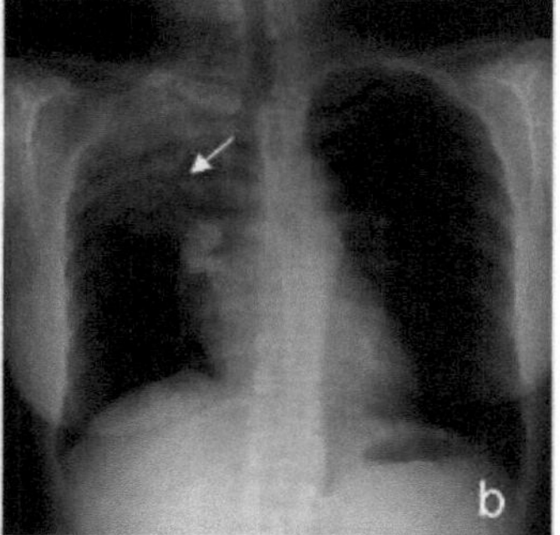

Fig. 60. Aerated bronchogram (a) diagram of bronchogram. Tubular clarity which bifurcates within an opacity. (b) Front chest X-ray. Tubular clarity bifurcating within an opacity (arrow).

3. Pathophysiology

The different densities of water and air give rise to the sign of an aerated bronchogram. This is a radiological sign resulting from the disappearance of the air normally contained in the pulmonary alveoli, this air being replaced by a liquid or by cells. The bronchus then becomes visible on standard radiology.

4. Causes

4.1. Pneumonia

Acute pneumonia is an acute infection of the lower airways characterised by inflammatory or even purulent damage to the lung parenchyma.

On imaging, systematised opacity with a watery tone, limited by a fissure, often impassable, containing an aerated bronchogram (fig. 61).

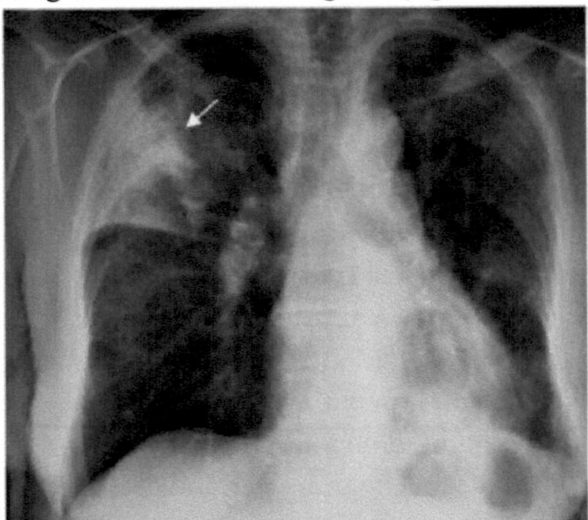

Fig. 61. Pneumonia. Radiograph of the front thorax. Opacity of watery tone, of the same density as the creur, systematised by the small scissure, containing an aerated bronchogram.

4.2. (Acute pulmonary edema

Butterfly wing opacities occur on either side of the two hili (fig. 62), affecting the base, but generally respecting the periphery of the lungs and the apices, the body of the butterfly being the mediastinum.

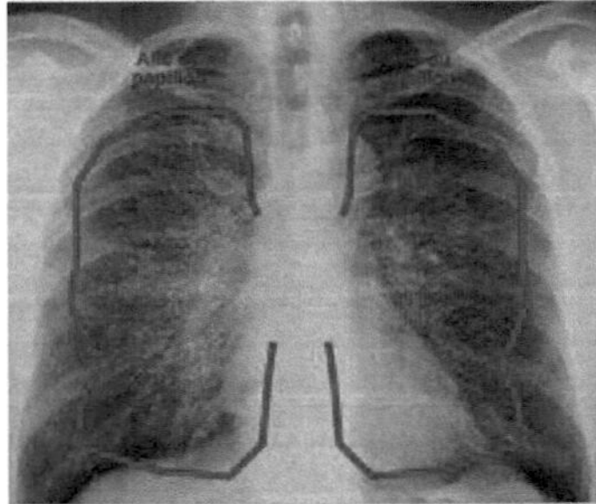

Fig. 62. Acute pulmonary oedema. Butterfly-shaped opacities.

4.3. Tuberculosis

Tuberculosis is an infectious disease caused by the bacterium Mycobacterium tuberculosis. On radiology, it presents as an opacity with an aerotic bronchogram (fig. 63).

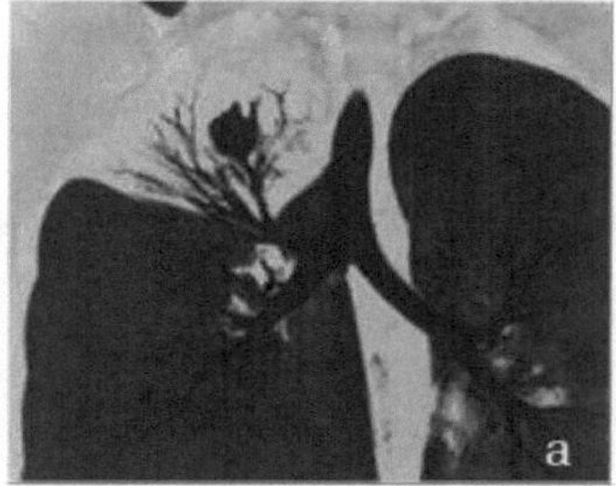

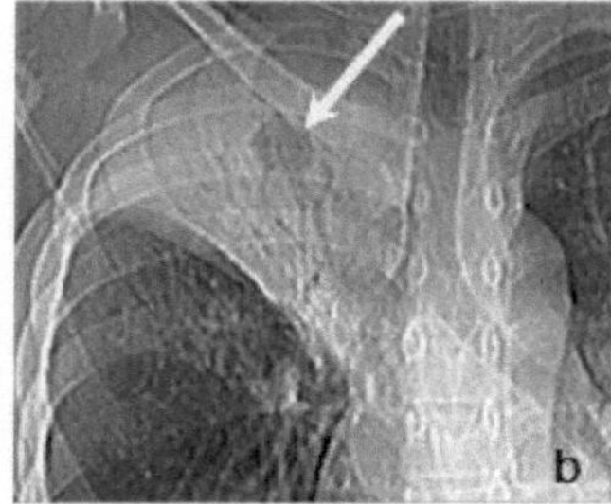

Fig. 63. Tuberculosis. Watery opacity with aerated bronchogram (a) frontal CT reconstruction, (b) standard frontal X-ray.

4.4. Other applications of the aerated bronchogram sign

Fig. 1. Adjoining bronchi indicate lobar or segmental atelectasis (fig. 64).

Fig. 2. Dilated bronchi indicate bronchiectasis (fig. 65).

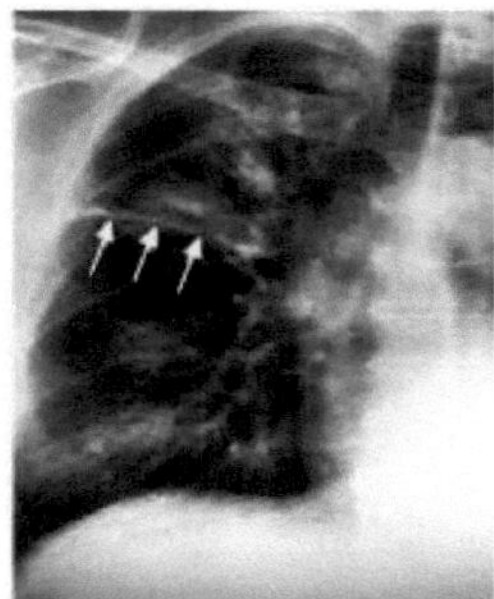

Fig. 64. Atelectasis. Band-like opacity, bronchi drawn together.

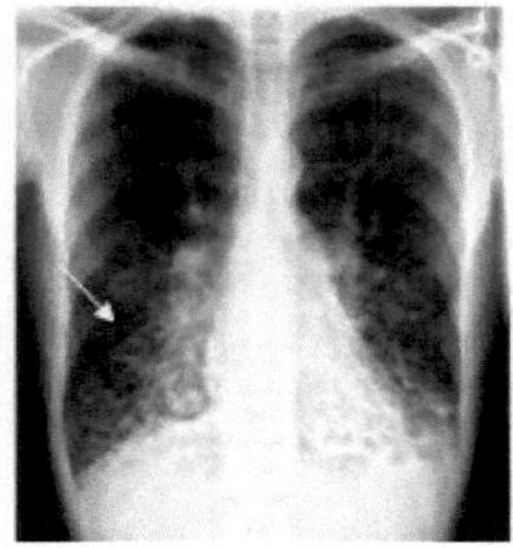

Fig. 65. Bronchiectasis. Dilatation of the bronchi, saccular hyperclartés.

5. Limits

A pulmonary lesion without an aeriform bronchogram, possibly related to :

- Bronchial tubes filled with secretions.
- Destroyed bronchial tubes.
- Congenitally absent bronchi.

If there is no sign of an aerated bronchogram in an opacity, the lesion is either pulmonary or extra-pulmonary.

Chapter 7

Lobar and segmental atelectasis

1. Definition

Partial or total volume reduction of the lung caused by a reduction in aeration. This term is preferred to collapsus, which should be reserved for massive atelectasis.

2. Mechanism

Three mechanisms leading to atelectasis:

- Obstruction.
- Compression.
- Shrinkage.

1.1. Obstructive atelectasis

Induced bronchial obstruction may be due to tumour or inflammatory stenosis, a foreign body, mucoid impaction or broncholithiasis due to major bronchial congestion.

Upstream of this blockage, the alveolar zone is no longer ventilated. Alveolar gas will gradually diffuse into the bloodstream, causing the alveolar zone to collapse and shrink, and therefore to be excluded from gas exchange. Obstruction may be single central or multiple peripheral.

1.1.1. Central obstruction

It may be of intrinsic or extrinsic origin.

- Intrinsic: bronchial cancer, foreign bodies, inflammatory bronchial diseases (tuberculosis).
- Extrinsic: masses, ADP, mediastinal tumour, aneurysm, or large creur.

1.1.2. Peripheral obstruction

Inflammatory exudates, mucus, etc.

1.2. Compression atelectasis

Due to extrinsic bronchial compression (adenopathy, mediastinal tumour, etc). It is said to be passive when there is compression by pleural effusion or another lesion.

Surfactant damage in acute respiratory distress syndrome also leads to atelectasis.

1.3. Retraction atelectasis

It may be due to the after-effects of tuberculosis or pulmonary fibrosis of various origins (silicosis).

3. Radiological signs of atelectasis

3.1. Direct Signs

- Displacement of the scissures bordering the affected lobe.
- Opacity.
- Silhouette sign.
- In the case of incomplete atelectasis: reduced aeration ± opacity, bronchial and vascular disorientation and compression.

• .1.1. Scissure displacement

The lung lobe is a pyramid with a pleural base and hilar apex containing bronchovascular arborisation fanning out from the hilum.

Peripheral base with two pleural layers, mediastinal face, scissural face and apex with limited mobility.

Atelectasis always tends to transform the lobar pyramid into a pleural-based, hilar-topped wafer, pressed against the mediastinum (fig. 66).

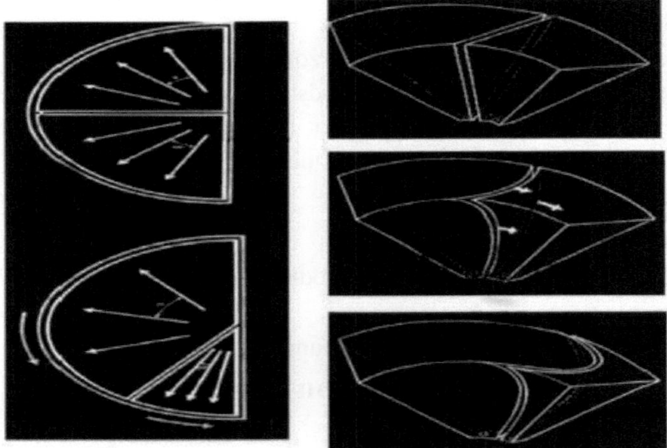

Fig. 66. Diagram showing the scissural displacement.

• .1.2. Opacity

Triangular opacity systematised in the lobe, with hilar apex and pleural base if non-ventilated collapse.

The opacity is detected on the frontal view, by comparing the two lungs and applying the silhouette sign (fig. 67).

On a normal profile view, each vertebral body appears blacker than its upper counterpart (thoracic vertebrae transparency gradient). In the case of an opacity, a loss of transparency gradient of the vertebrae "Spine sign" will be observed (fig. 68).

In most cases, there is a reduction in aeration associated with opacity with vascular and bronchial displacements (fig. 69).

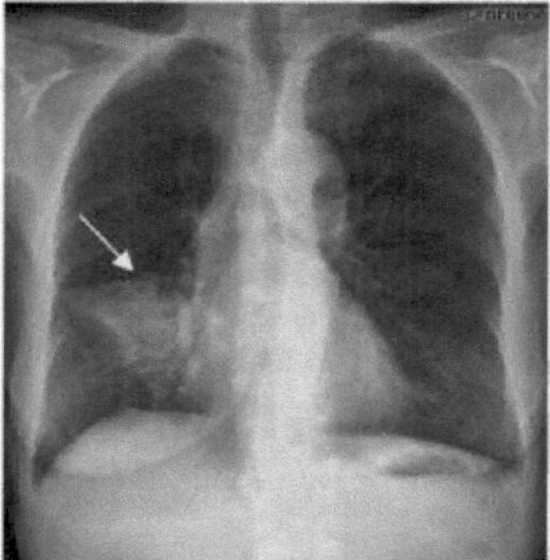

Fig. 67. Opacity on frontal view. Triangular opacity systematized by the small scissure of the middle lobe (arrow), erasing the right edge of the creur (silhouette sign).

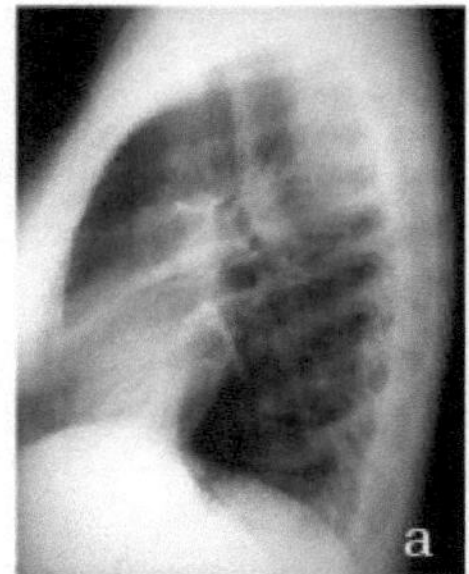

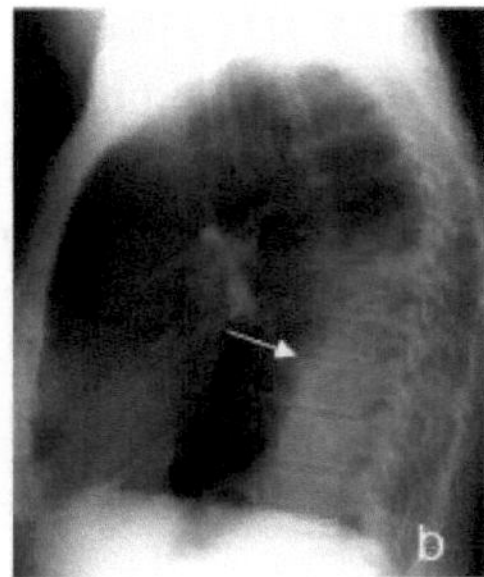

Fig. 68. Opacity on lateral view. (a) Profile without abnormality, with gradient of transparency of the vertebrae. (b) Posterior opacity, positive spine sign (arrow).

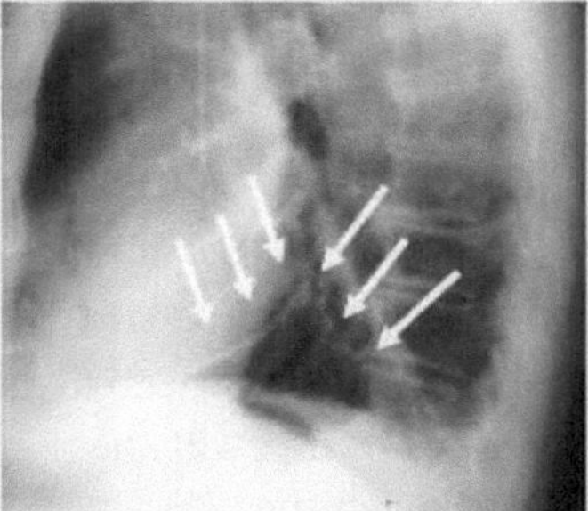

Fig. 69. Decreased pulmonary aeration and vascular and bronchial displacement.

3.2. Indirect signs (fig. 70)

3.2.1. Moving hilariously.

3.2.2. Unilateral elevation of the diaphragmatic dome.

3.2.3. Mediastinal displacement (trachea, creili j.

3.2.4. Loss of volume in the ipsilateral hemithorax.

3.2.5. Compensatory hyperinflation of the healthy lobes.

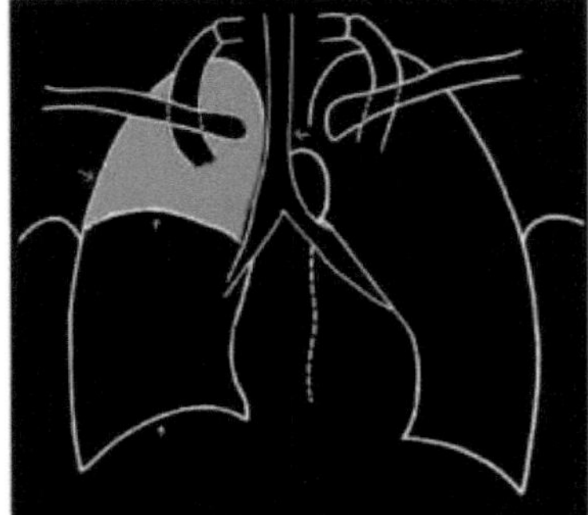

Fig. 70. Indirect signs of atelectasis.

3.2.6. Hilary displacement

This is the most important indirect sign. Normally, in 97% of normal individuals, the left hilum is higher than the right, and in 3% of normal individuals, the hilums are at the same level (fig. 71).

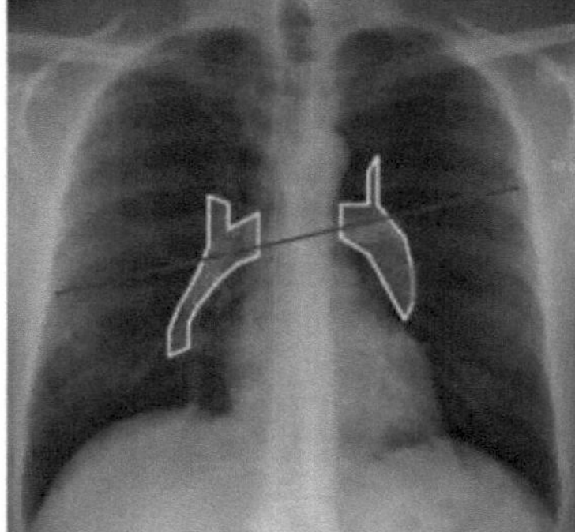

Fig. 71. The left hilum higher than the right.

3.2.7. Elevation of the diaphragmatic dome

Ascension of the diaphragmatic dome homolateral to the atelectasis.
The diaphragmatic domes are asymmetric, with the right diaphragmatic dome normally 1 to 2 cm higher than the left (fig. 72).

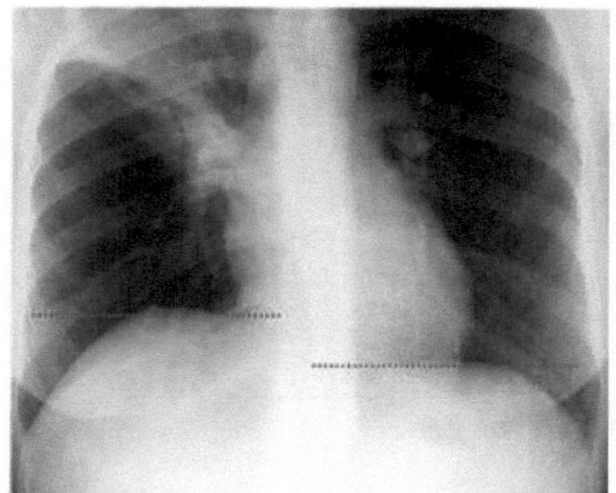

Fig. 72. The right diaphragmatic dome is higher than the left.

3.2.8. Mediastinal displacement

Displacement of the trachea towards atelectasis. The creur is rarely deviated; it requires a significant loss of volume (fig. 73).

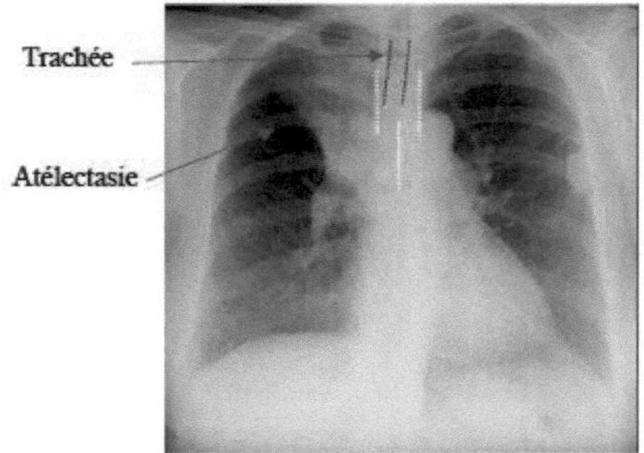

Trachea Atelectasis

Fig. 73. Tracheal shift atelectasis.

3.2.9. Compensatory hyperinflation

Compensatory hyperclarity of the parenchyma of the healthy lobes (fig.74).

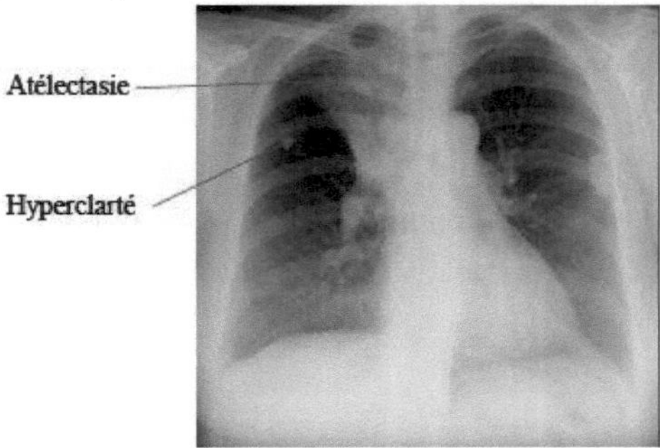

Atelectasis Hyperclarity

Fig. 74. Retractile opacity of the right upper lobe associated with compensatory hyperclarity of a homolateral lobe of the lung.

3.3. Associated signs

Golden's "inverted S" sign is a hilar mass with loss of volume resulting in central convexity and peripheral concavity at level of the scissure (fig. 75).

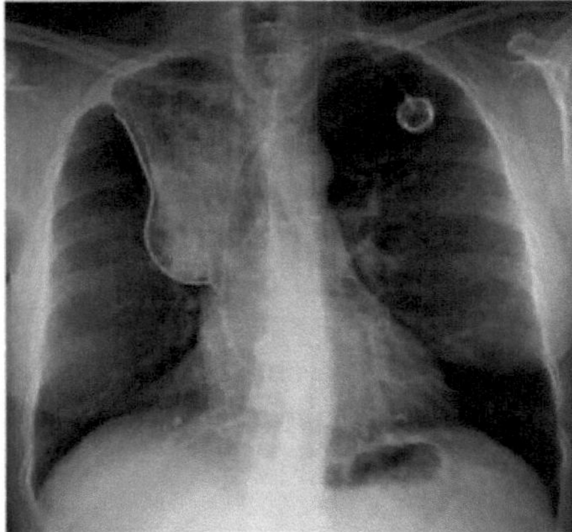

Fig. 75. Golden sign.

4. Lobe atelectasis

4.1. Atelectasis of the right upper lobe

4.1.1. Direct signs

4.1.1.1 Face

- Clear opacity in the right upper region (triangular opacity with hilar apex).
- Upward and medial displacement of the lesser scissure (fig. 76).

4.1.1.2 Profile

The small scissure and the upper half of the large scissure will move upwards until they meet (closing a book) (fig.77).

4.1.2. Indirect signs

- Right wing same level or higher than left wing.
- Deviation of the trachea to the right.
- Elevation of the right diaphragmatic dome.
- Hyperclarity of the right middle and lower lobes compared with the left lung.

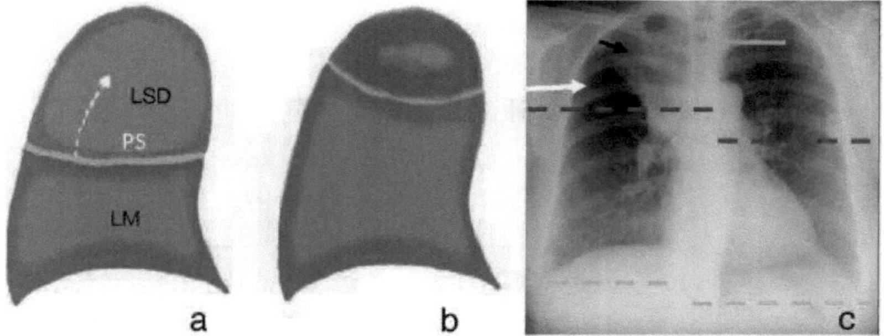

Fig. 76. Frontal atelectasis of the right upper lobe. (a+b) Diagrams of displacement of the small fissure (PS) to form a right upper lobar opacity. (c) Standard radiograph. Right upper lobar opacity (black arrow), tracheal deviation to the right (green arrow), hyperclarity of the middle lobe (white arrow), right hilum higher than the left hilum and elevation of the right diaphragmatic dome.

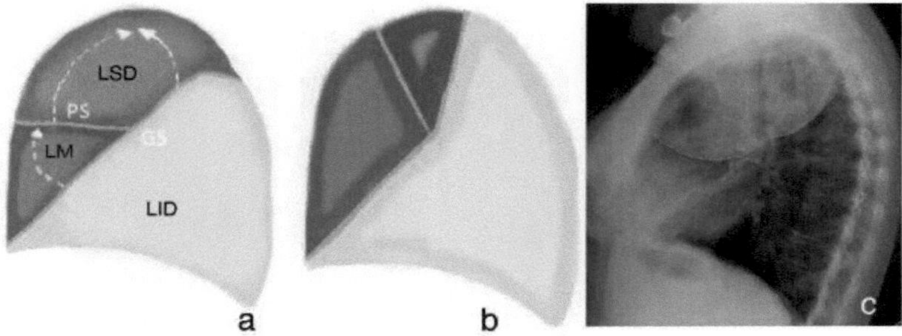

Fig. 77. Right upper lobe atelectasis in profile. (a+b) Right lung diagrams in profile, (c) standard radiograph in profile. Displacement of the scissures in atelectasis of the right upper lobe in profile. Small fissure (PS). Large fissure (GS).

4.2. Left upper lobe atelectasis

4.2.1. Direct signs

4.2.1.1 Face

- Homogeneous peri- and supra-hilar opacity on the left (fig. 78).

4.2.1.2 Profile

- Large scissure drawn upwards and forwards (antero-superior)
- The opacity is parallel and pressed against the anterior chest wall (fig.79).

4.2.2. Indirect signs

- Elevation of the left hilum.
- Deviation of the trachea to the left.

- Elevation of the left diaphragmatic dome.
- Hyperclarity of the left lower lobe.

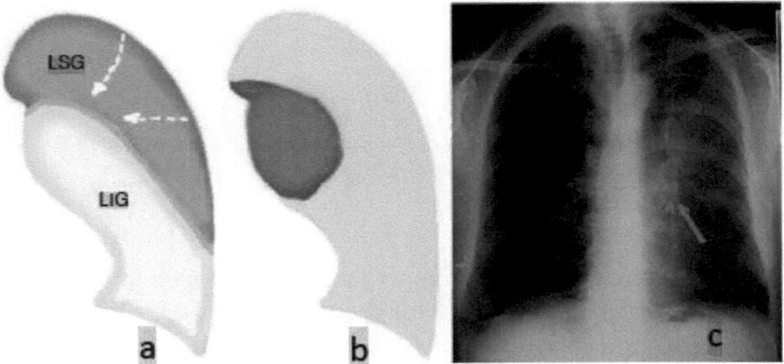

Fig. 78. Front view of left upper lobe atelectasis. (a+b) Front view of left lung, (c) Front view of standard X-ray. Peri-hilar opacity (arrow).

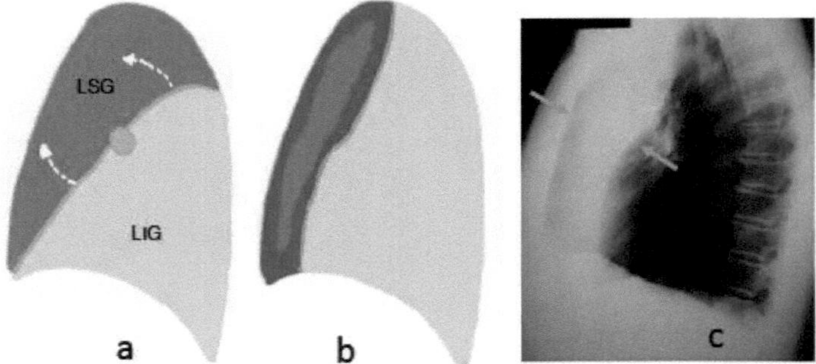

Fig. 79. Left upper lobe atelectasis in profile. (a+b) Lung diagrams in profile, (c) standard X-ray in profile. Opacity parallel and flat against the anterior chest wall (arrows).

4.3. Atelectasis of the middle lobe / lingula

4.3.1. Direct signs

The lesser and greater scissures are brought closer together in an inferomedial and superomedial direction respectively, until an opacity obliterating the right edge of the heart is obtained on the front and a linear opacity in a posteroanterior and craniocaudal direction from the right hilum is obtained on the side (figs. 80 and 81).

4.3.2. Indirect signs

- No significant displacement of the hilum.
- No significant displacement of the homolateral trachea.
- Hyperclarity of the right upper lobe compared with the left lung.

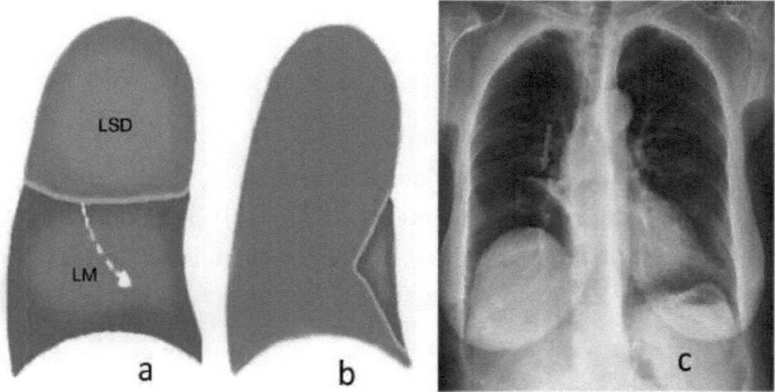

Fig. 80. Front view of middle lobe atelectasis (a+b) Front lung diagrams, (c) Front standard X-ray. Opacity obliterating the right edge of the creur (arrow).

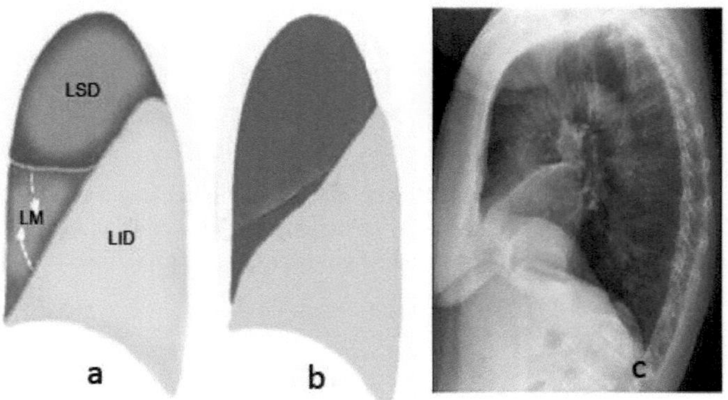

Fig. 81. Middle lobe atelectasis in profile. (a+b) Lung diagrams in profile, (c) Standard profile X-ray. Anterior linear opacity (arrows).

4.4. Atelectasis of the right lower lobe

4.4.1. Direct signs

4.4.1.1 Face

Displacement of the superior-external part of the greater scissure in an inferomedial direction. Its lateral part turns backwards to become tangent to the X-rays. More severe atelectasis leads to the formation of a triangular infra hilar opacity obliterating the edge of the diaphragm and the paravertebral interface (fig. 82).

4.4.1.2 Profile

The two upper and lower portions the greater scissure descend as they turn backwards to form a conical opacity whose apex is hilar and whose base is the posterior and inferior part of the thoracic wall and the posterior part of the hemidiaphragm (fig. 83).

4.4.2. Indirect signs

- Lower displacement of the right hilum.
- Tracheal shift towards the homolateral side.
- Elevation of the right hemidiaphragm.
- Hyperclarity of the middle right upper lobe compared with the left lung.

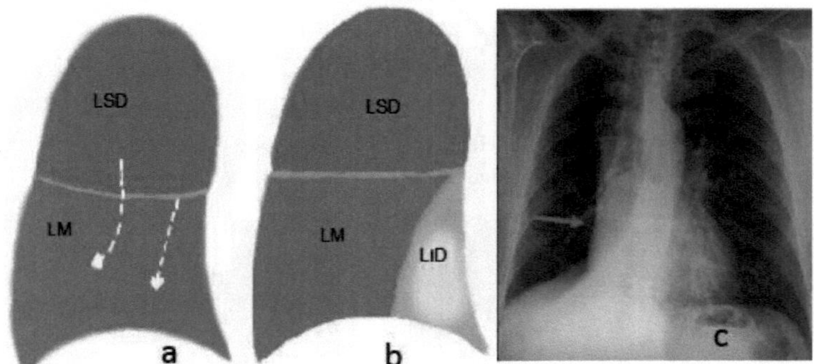

Fig. 82. Frontal atelectasis of the right lower lobe. (a+b) Frontal lung diagrams, (c) Frontal standard X-ray. Triangular infrahilar opacity obliterating the edge of the diaphragm and the paravertebral interface, does not obliterate the right edge of the heart (arrow).

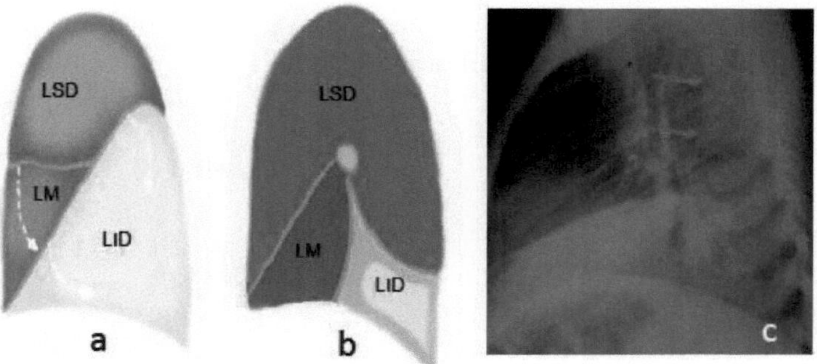

Fig. 83. Right lower lobe atelectasis in profile. (a+b) Lung diagrams in profile, (c) Standard profile X-ray. Conical opacity with a hilar apex and a base at the posterior and inferior part of the chest wall (arrows).

4.5. Left lower lobe atelectasis

4.5.1. Direct signs

4.5.1.1 Face

Clear opacity in the left medial and inferior zone (fig.84).

4.5.1.2 Profile

Large scissure drawn downwards and backwards (fig. 85).

4.5.2. Indirect signs

- Lower displacement of the left hilum.
- Tracheal shift towards the homolateral side.
- Elevation of the left hemidiaphragm.
- Hyperclarity of the left upper lobe compared with the right lung.

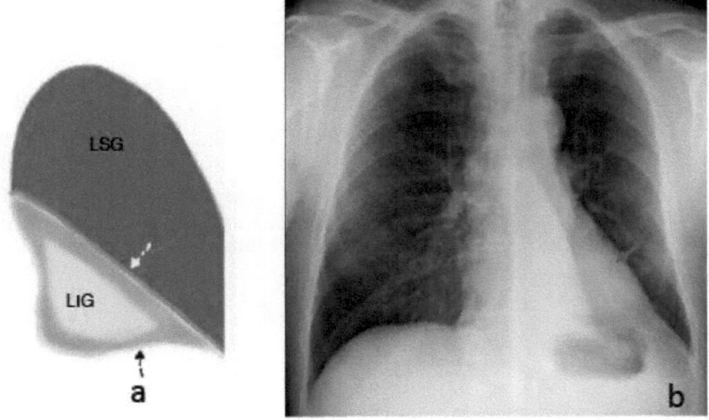

Fig. 84. Frontal atelectasis of the left lower lobe. (a+b) Frontal lung diagrams

, (c) Frontal standard X-ray. Opacity of the left lower and medial zone, not obliterating the left edge of the heart (arrow).

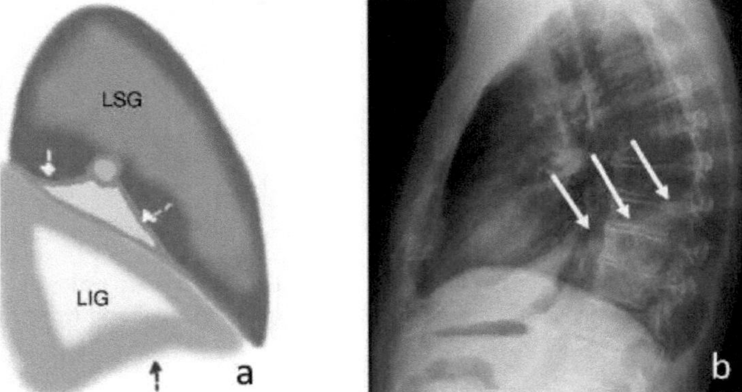

Fig. 85. Left lower lobe atelectasis in profile. (a+b) Lung diagrams in profile, (c) Standard X-ray in profile. Triangular opacity with a hilar apex and a base at the posterior and inferior part of the chest wall (red arrow). The greater fissure is drawn downwards and backwards (white arrows).

5. Atelectasis of an entire lung

On imaging, this manifests itself as an opacity of the pulmonary hemichamber, with protrusion of the normal lung into the affected hemi thorax and attraction of the mediastinum towards the affected side, unlike a large pleural effusion which pushes the mediastinum towards the healthy side (fig.86).

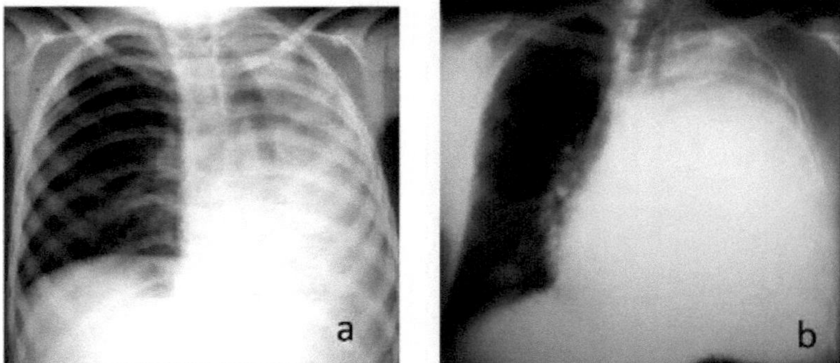

Fig. 86. Front radiograph: (a) Atelectasis of the entire lung draws in the mediastinum. (b) Large pleural effusion draws in the mediastinum.

Reference

1. Adams G, Wein B, Keulers B, Stargardt A, Guenther RW. Quality of intensive care chest imaging: comparison of conventional phosphorous plak system with conventional radiography in bedside imaging. Radiology 1989;173(P):402.
2. Austin JH. The left minor fissure. Radiology 1996;161:433-6.
3. Armstrong WB, Netterville JL. Anatomy of the larynx, trachea and bronchi. Otolaryngol Clin North Am 1995;28:685-704.
4. Brun AL. Alveolar syndrome. EMC - Radiology and Medical Imaging - cardiovascular - thoracic - cervical 2014;9(2):1-9 [Article 32-360-A-10].
5. Bachman AL, Teixidor HS. The posterior tracheal band a reflector of local superior mediastinal abnormality. Br J Radiol 1975; 48: 352-359
6. Boyden EA, Hartman JF. Analysis of variations in the bronchopulmonary segments of the left upper lobe of 50 lungs. AmJ Anat 1946; 79:321-60.
7. Boyden EA, Scannell JG. An analysis of variations in the bronchovascular pattern of the right upper lobe of 50 lungs. Am J Anat 1948; 82:27-73.
8. Boyden EA, Hamre CJ. An analysis of variations in the bronchovascular pattern of the middle lobe in 50 dissected and 20 injected lungs. J Thorac Surg 1951;21:172-88.
9. Boyden EA. In: Segmental anatomy of the lung: a study of the pattern of the segmental bronchi and selected pulmonary vessels. New York: McGraw-Hill; 1955. p. 23-32.
10. Babichev EA, Baru SE, Khabakhpashev AG, Kolachev GM, Ponomarev OA, Savinov GA, et al. Digital radiographic device baseon NWPC with improved spatial resolution. Nucl Instrd Methods Phys Res 1992;A323:49-53.
11. Berkmen T, Berkmen YM, Austin JH. Accessory fissures of the upper lobe of the left lung: CT plain film appearance. AJR Am J Roentgenol 1994;162:1287-93.
12. Breatnach E, Abbott GC, Fraser RG. Dimensions of the normal human trachea. AJR Am J Roentgenol 1984;142:903Felson B. Chest roentgenology. Philadelphia: WB Saunders, 1973
13. Beigelman C, Meunier C, Trogrlic S. Radioanatomy of the thorax. In: Jeanbourquin D, editor. Imagerie thoracique de l'adulte. Paris: Masson; 2003. p. 7-57.
14. Beigelman C. Tomodensitometry. In: Grenier P, editor. Imagerie thoracique de l'adulte. Paris: Médecine-Sciences Flammarion; 1996. p. 51-105.
15. Coussement A, Padovani B. Lateral incidence of the thorax. Cours perfectionnement post- universitaire. Journées françaises de radiologie, Paris, November 1997
16. Chotas HG, Floyd CE, Ravin CE. Evaluation of a digital chest radiography system uses a selenium detector. Radiology 1995;195: 264-70.
17. Cooper C, Moss AA, Buy JN, Stark DD. CT appearance of the normal inferior pulmonary ligament. AJR Am J Roentgenol 1983;141:237-40.
18. Chotas HG, Dobbins JT, Ravin CE. Principles of digital radiography with large area, electronically readable detectors: a review of the basics. Radiology 1999;210:595-9.
19. Dubois De Montreynaud J.M., Lecture accélérée de la radiographique thoracique, 2nd edition, Maloine, Paris, 1996.
20. Daniel Anthoine, Jean-Claude Humbert. La radiologie thoracique standard (face and profiles), Atlas de pathologie thoracique (2007).
21. Debray MP, Bancal C, Dombret MC. Normal and pathological non-tumorous pleura. EMC - Radiology and medical imaging - cardiovascular - thoracic - cervical 2013;8(3):1- 15 [Article 32-520-A-10].

22. Debray MP, Bancal C, Dombret MC. Normal and pathological non-tumoral Pl\®vre. EMC - Radiology and Medical Imaging - Cardiovascular - Thoracic - Cervical 2013;8(3):1-15 [Article 32-520-A-10].
23. Dobbins JT, Samei E, Chotas HG, Warp RJ, Baydush AH, Floyd CE, et al. Chest radiography: optimization of X-ray spectrum for cesium iodide amorphous silicon flat panel detector. Radiology 2003;226: 221-30.
24. Frija J., De Bazelaire C., Mathieu O., Zagdanski A-M., DeKerviler E., Guide de lecture à partir de l'anatomie radiologique du thorax, Journées Françaises de Radiologie 2004 - Formation Médicale Continue N° 55.
25. Foote GA, Meredith HC. The silhouette sign and the inferior vena cava. Radiology 1979; 133: 583-585.
26. Frija J, Schmit P, Katz M, Vadrot D, Laval-Jeantet M. Computed tomography of the pulmonary fissures. Normal anatomy. J Comput Assist Tomogr 1982; 6: 1069-1074
27. Fraser RG, Pare JA, Pare PD, Fraser RS, Genereux GP. The normal chest. In: Diagnosis diseases of the chest. Philadelphia:WB Saunders; 1988.
28. Frija J, de Géry S, Lallouet F, Guermazi A, Zagdanski AM, de Kerviller E. Digital chest radiography: equipment, image processing, limitations. J Radiol 2001;82:1045-53.
29. Floyd Jr. CE, Baker JA, Chotas HG, Delong DM, Ravin CE. Selenium based digital radiography of the chest: radiologist preference compared with film screen radiographs. AJR Am J Roentgenol 1995;165:1353-8.
30. Felson B., Weinstein A. S., Spitz H. B., Principes de la radiologie du thorax, 2 volume edition, Delachaux & Niestel, Neuchatel- Paris, 1979.
31. Fischer MS. Significance of a visible major fissure on the frontal chest radiograph. AJR Am J Roentgenol 1981;137:477-80.
32. GlazerHS, MolinaPL, SiegelMJ,Sagel SS. High-attenuation mediastinal masses on unenhanced CT. AJR Am J Roentgenol 1991; 156: 45-50
33. Giron J, Coussement A, Sans N, Fajadet P, Sénac JP, Durand Get al. Incidence latéraleduthorax : " leprofil ". EncyclMed Chir (Elsevier, Paris), Radiodiagnostic-Coeur-Poumon, 32-330-A15, 1997: 1-28
34. Giron J, Sénac JP. Manual of thoracic imaging. Le profil. Montpellier: Sauramps Medical, 1995.
35. Goodwin JD, Tarver RD. Accessory fissures of the lung. AJR Am J Roentgenol 1985; 144: 39-47
36. Grenier P, Guilbeau JC. Chest radiography: normal findings. In: Grenier P, editor. Imagerie thoracique de l'adulte. Paris: Médecine-Sciences Flammarion; 1996. p. 9-25.
37. Grenier P. Imagerie thoracique de l'adulte. Paris: Médecine-Sciences Flammarion; 1996.
38. Grenier P. Radiographie du thorax : les syndromes radiologiques.niveau PCEM2 - EIA appareil respiratoire 2002 - 2003
39. Godwin JD, Tarver RD. Accessory fissures of the lung. AJR Am J Roentgenol 1985;144:39- 47.
40. HeitzmanER,LaneEJ,HammackDB,RimmierLJ. Radiological evaluation of the aortic-pulmonic window. Radiology 1975; 116: 513-51.
41. Hayashi K, Aziz A, Ashizawa K, Hayashi H, Nagaoki K, Otsuji H. Radiographic andCTappearances of the major fissures. Radiographics 2001;21:861-74.-6. 1984.
42. Haskin PH, Goodman LR. Normal trachea bifurcation angle: a reassessment. AJR Am J Roentgenol 1982;139:879-82.

43. Jackson CL, Huber JF. Correlated applied anatomy of bronchial tree and lungs with a system of nomenclature. Dis Chest 1943;9:319-26.
44. Jeanbourquin D., Lahutte M., Teriitehau C., El Kharras A., Geffroy Y., Minvielle F., Normal lung. EMC (Elsevier SAS, Paris), Radiodiagnostic - Creur-poumon, 32-330-A-10, 2006.
45. Jardin M, Rémy J. Segmental bronchovascular anatomy of the lower lobes: CT analysis. AJR Am J Roentgenol 1986;147:457-68.
46. Jeanbourquin D, Hazebroucq V, Beroud P, Attia M, Cordoliani YS, Cosnard G. CT visualisation of segmental bronchi. Med Armees 1987;15:457-68.
47. Kramer R, Glass A. Bronchoscopic localization of lung abcess. Ann Otol Laryngol 1932;14:1210-20.
48. Kido S, Ikezeo J, Takeuchi N, Kondoh H, Tomiyama N, Joko T, et al. Interpretation of subtle interstitial lung abnormalities: conventional versus storage phosphor radiography. Radiology 1993;187:527-33.
49. Kundel HL, GefterW, Aronchik J, Miller Jr.W, Habatu H,Withfill CH, et al. Accuracy of bedside chest hard copy screen film versus hard and soft copy computed radiographs in a medical intensive care unit: receiver operating characteristic analysis. Radiology 1997;205: 859-63.
50. Kalifa G, Charpak Y, Maccia C, Fery-Lemonnier E, Bloch J, Boussard JM, et al. Evaluation of low dose digital X-ray device: first dosimetric and clinical results in children. Pediatr Radiol 1998;28: 557-61.
51. Kent EM, Blades B. The surgical anatomy of the pulmonary lobes. J Thorac Surg 1942;12:18- 30.
52. Lacombe P, Chatel A, Latouche D, Bigot JM, Helenon C. La région aortico-pulmonaire.Anatomieet anatomie radiologique normale et pathologique. Feuillets Radiol1979;114: 409-408
53. Landay MJ. Azygos vein abutting the posterior wall of the right main and upper lobe bronchi: a normal CT variant. AJR Am J Roentgenol 1983;140:461-2.
54. Monnier J.P., Tubiana J.M., Cahier de radiologie, tome 3: le poumon, Masson, Paris,
55. Mathieu Lederlin. sV©mV©iological thoracic radiology. Main syndromes. CHU Rennes.
56. Maccia C, Ducou Le Pointe H, Fery-Lemonnier E, Nadeau X, Montagne JP, Charpentier E, et al. Photostimulable plates or conventional films for bed-side lung imaging in paediatric radiology? A comparative study of image quality and patient dose. J Radiol 1996;77:1129-34.
57. Medlar EM. Variation in interlobar fissures. AJR Am J Roentgenol 1947;57:723-5.
58. Naidich JB, Naidich TP, Hyman RA, Schwartz K, Goldman MA, Pudlowski RM. The big rib sign localisation of basal pulmonary pathology in lateral projection utilizing differential magnification of the two hemithoraces. Radiology 1979; 131: 1-8
59. Piver D, Bisseret D, Bertrand G, Sans N, Brillet PY. Bronchial syndrome. EMC - Radiology and medical imaging - cardiovascular - thoracic - cervical 2016;11(4):1-16 [Article 32-360-C-10].
60. Palayew MJ. The tracheo-esophageal stripe and the posterior tracheal band. Radiology 1979; 132: 11-13.
61. Proto AV, Speckman JM. The left lateral radiograph of the chest (part one). Med Radiogr Photogr 1979; 55: 30-76.
62. Proto AV, Speckman JM. The left lateral radiograph of the chest (part two). Med Radiogr Photogr 1980; 56: 38-64.

63. Proto AV, Ball Jr. JB. The superolateral major fissure. AJR Am J Roentgenol 1983;140:431- 7.
64. Putman GE, Curtis AM, Westfried M, McLoud TC. Thickening of the posterior tracheal stripe. A sign of squamous cell carcinoma of the esophagus. Radiology 1976; 121: 533-536.
65. Prakash UB, Fontana RS. Functional classification of bronchial carinae. Chest 1984;86:770- 2.
66. Raymond Capdeville. Introduction to pulmonary radiology. Traité de Radiodiagnostic III - Creur-poumon: 32- 330-A-05 (1995).
67. Raasch BN, Carsky EW, Lane EJ, O'Callaghan JP, Heitzman ER.Radiographicanatomyoftheinterlobar fissures.Astudy of 100 specimens. AJR Am J Roentgenol 1982 ; 138 :1043-1049.
68. Remy J, Lemaitre L, Smith M. Die Topographisch-RadiologischeAnatomiedesRechtensubkarinarenundretrobronchialen Pulmonalen Recessus. Radiologe1981; 21: 324-329.
69. Rowlands JA. Digital X-ray systems based on amorphous selenium. AJR Am J Roentgenol 1996;167:409-11.
70. Rowlands JA, Zho W, Blevis IM, Waechter DF, Huang Z. Flat panel digital radiology with amorphous selenium and active matrix readout. Radiographics 1997;17:753-60.
71. Raasch BN, Carski EW, Lane EJ. Radiographic anatomy of the interlobar fissures: a study of 100 specimens. AJR Am J Roentgenol 1982;138:1043-9.
72. Raasch BN, Carsky EW, Lane EJ, O'Callaghan JP, Heitzman ER. Radiographic anatomy of the interlobar fissures: a study of 10 specimens. AJR Am J Roentgenol 1982;138:1043-9.
73. Rost RC, Proto AV. Inferior pulmonary ligament: computed tomography appearance. Radiology 1983;148:179-83.
74. Shields JE, Holtz S. The retrotracheal space. Radiology 1976; 120: 19-23
75. Szamosi A. Anterior border of the left atrium on conventional heart films. Acta Radiol Diagn 1978; 19: 57-63
76. Schaefer-Prokop CM, Prokop M, Schmidt A, Neitzel U, Galanski M. Selenium radiography versus storage phosphor and conventional radiography in the detection of simulated chest lesions. Radiology 1996;201:45-50.
77. Scannell JG, Boyden EA. A study of variations of the bronchopulmonary segments in the right upper lobe (in 13 injected specimen). J Thorac Surg 1948;17:303-8.
78. Sealy WC, Connally SR, Dalton ML. Naming the bronchopulmonary segments and the development of pulmonary surgery. Ann Thorac Surg 1993;55:184-8.
79. Tran R, Montaudon M, Latrabe V and Laurent F. Mediastinal syndrome. Encycl Méd Chir (Editions Scientifiques et Médicales Elsevier SAS, Paris, all rights reserved), Radiodiagnostic - Coeur-Poumon, 32-360-P-10, 2001, 19 p.
80. Uffman M, Neitzel U, Prokop M, Kabalan N,Weber M, Herold CJ, et al. Flat panel detector chest radiography: effect of tube voltage on image quality. Radiology 2005;235:642-50.
81. Vincent J. Étude anatomo-radiologique de l'incidence d profil du thorax: résultats normaux et applications pathologiques. [thesis], Grenoble, 1976
82. Van Heesewijk HP, Neitzel U, Van der Graaf Y, de Valois JC, Felberg MA. Digital chest imaging with a selenium detector: comparison with conventional radiography for vizualization of specific anatomic regions of the chest. AJRAm J Roentgenol 1995;165:535-40.

83. Van Heesewijk HP,Van der GraafY, deValois JC, Felberg SA. Effect of dose reduction on digital chest imaging using a selenium detector: study of detecting simulated diffuse interstitial pulmonary disease. AJR Am J Roentgenol 1996;167:403-8.
84. Wescott J, Ferguson D. The right pulmonary artery. Left atrial axis line (a method for measuring left atrial size on lateral chest radiographs). Radiology 1976; 118: 265-267
85. Whalen JP, Meyers MA, Oliphant M, Caragol WJ, Evans JA. The retrosternal line: a new sign of an anterior mediastinal mass. AJR Am J Roentgenol 1973; 117: 861-862.
86. Whalen JP, Oliphant M, Evans JA. Anterior extrapleural line superior extension. Radiology 1975; 115: 525-531.
87. Yamashita H. Roentgenologic anatomy of the lung. Stuttgart: Thieme Verlag; 1978.

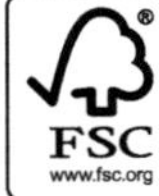

MIX
Papier aus verantwortungsvollen Quellen
Paper from responsible sources
FSC® C105338

Printed by Books on Demand GmbH, Norderstedt / Germany